Clinical Management of Overweight and Obesity

T0297460

Paolo Sbraccia • Enzo Nisoli • Roberto Vettor
Editors

Clinical Management of Overweight and Obesity

Recommendations of the Italian Society of Obesity (SIO)

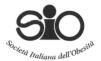

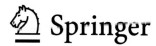

Editors
Paolo Sbraccia
Department of Systems Medicine
Medical School
University of Rome "Tor Vergata"
Rome
Italy

Roberto Vettor
Center for the Study and the Integrated
Treatment of Obesity
University of Padua
Padua
Italy

Enzo Nisoli
Department of Medical Biotechnology
and Translational Medicine
University of Milan
Milan
Italy

Based on the document "Standard Italiani per la Cura dell'Obesità", published online 2012
by Società Italiana dell'Obesità

ISBN 978-3-319-24530-0   ISBN 978-3-319-24532-4   (eBook)
DOI 10.1007/978-3-319-24532-4

Library of Congress Control Number: 2015957407

Springer Cham Heidelberg New York Dordrecht London
© Springer International Publishing Switzerland 2016

Printed on acid-free paper

Springer International Publishing AG Switzerland is part of Springer Science+Business Media
(www.springer.com)

Preface

It is with great pleasure that we present *Clinical Management of Overweight and Obesity: Recommendations of the Italian Society of Obesity (SIO)*.

This book of guidelines is the result of efforts by a group of Italian experts in the treatment of obesity. Responsibility for individual sections has rested with, Luca Busetto, Barbara Cresci, Massimo Cuzzolaro, Lorenzo M. Donini, Pierpaolo De Feo, Annunziata Lapolla, Lucio Lucchin, Claudio Maffeis, Fabrizio Pasanisi, Carlo Rotella, Ferruccio Santini, and Mauro Zamboni. To everybody, who has been involved in the project, but especially to those just mentioned, we express our heartfelt thanks.

The book addresses the obesity problem in diverse circumstances from pregnancy to old age, ending with a treatment algorithm that hopefully will lead over the years to new and more effective therapeutic tools. There is no doubting the need!

The book is intended as a guide, based on scientific evidence. It should be useful not only to those who are at the forefront in caring for people with obesity but also to the many other specialists whose encounters with obese patients and their problems are becoming ever more frequent.

Nevertheless, launching these guidelines, in which we take much pride, we would also like to draw attention to some particular considerations and possible caveats.

In recent years, there has been a significant increase in the publication of guidelines for clinical practice, even if there is a growing awareness that the mere publication of a guide does not guarantee that what is being suggested as best practice translates effectively into the clinical choices made on a daily basis. The continuing need for major revisions to clinical practice reflects the gap that can exist between advice in guidelines and what actually happens in daily routine. On the other hand, there is a danger that is potentially creeping into the relationship between the publication of guidelines and clinical practice a danger resulting from the accelerating turnover of knowledge in specific sectors.

Guidelines are part of the decision-making process, offering the support of a shared body of knowledge and operational choices tested in respect of efficacy and safety. They proceed from shared theoretical assumptions and solid experimental conclusions (clinical trials, validated meta-analysis) and propose solutions, decisions, and behaviors widely accepted and adopted by the scientific community. It is in this context that mistakes can arise. Those who use established knowledge and apply codified rules to clarify, for example, a diagnostic problem or to decide on a particular course of therapy may fall short of their objective for a whole range of reasons. For example, they may not have used the concepts best suited to the case in hand. Alternatively, they may not have employed the concepts and/or techniques available, or they may have resorted to an inappropriate rule or regulation, and so on. The guidelines have been laid down precisely to bring order to a massive body of knowledge, often not consistent, centering around specific topics so as to classify and standardize choices in clinical practice and so reduce operational errors. At least as regards the limited period of time in which they were proposed, they are the result of a theoretical construct deemed true in that it is based on the probability that the observed data match the body of theoretical assumptions considered highly likely by the scientific community.

At a historical moment when there is a potential discrepancy between the tremendous acceleration in knowledge turnover and guideline publication, guidelines may already be obsolete by the time they come to be defined and applied.

In effect, "evidence-based medicine" and clinical guidelines rarely provide the definitive answer to clinical problems; rather, they are subject to many changes that are all the more drastic given the pace of the emergence of new knowledge. For these reasons, we intend to continually update these guidelines, which will always be available on the two organizations' websites.

In addition, although the book does not address the complex issue of complications arising from obesity, it is also appropriate to distinguish between generic clinical decisions manageable through the guidelines and complex decisions typical for the elderly patient with multiple pathologies or with a pathology like obesity that brings with it a wide range of other conditions, which these days require the doctor to be capable of directly managing the scientific knowledge available (knowledge management).

The key to understanding how the world works is to question its nature, being always ready to give up previous ideas if the answers contradict what we think.

It is in this spirit that *Clinical Management of Overweight and Obesity: Recommendations of the Italian Society of Obesity (SIO)* is published. The drafting of these guidelines, as stated above, is and will be founded on a continuous collaboration with those who feel a need to revise, correct, supplement, and implement these operational suggestions. In this contex, we would like to cite the words that spoken by Winston Churchill in a rather more dramatic predicament, but which seem eminently applicable here, too: "This is not the end, not even the beginning of the end. But it is perhaps the end of the beginning."

The Editors,
Paolo Sbraccia
Enzo Nisoli
Roberto Vettor

Introduction

Although it was only in 1950 that obesity was introduced into the international classification of diseases (currently code ICD-10 E66), it has already reached epidemic proportions before the end of the century, becoming one of the leading causes of death and disability worldwide. In 2014, 2 billion adults (over 20 years of age) were overweight, and it was estimated that 500 million adults worldwide were obese: over 200 million men and nearly 300 million women. About 65% of the world's population currently live in countries where overweight and obesity kill more than underweight ones. The number of people afflicted is growing without any decline, and more than 40 million children under 5 years old proved to be overweight in 2010. According to the WHO, "Obesity is one of the greatest public health challenges of the twenty-first century. Its prevalence has tripled in many countries of the WHO European Region since the 1980s, and the numbers of those affected continue to rise at an alarming rate. In addition to causing various physical disabilities and psychological problems, excess weight drastically increases a person's risk of developing a number of noncommunicable diseases (NCDs), including cardiovascular disease, cancer and diabetes."

The recommendation to reduce body weight in overweight or obese individuals is therefore mandatory. However, long-term treatment is a challenging task and requires an integrated approach using all the available instruments in a complementary way, drawing on diverse professional skills but all sharing the same therapeutic objective.

The first aim of *Clinical Management of Overweight and Obesity: Recommendations of the Italian Society of Obesity (SIO)* is to serve as a practical point of reference for all the many professionals responsible for treating people with obesity; however, this is also for researchers, students, and the patients themselves who intend to, in the context of a therapeutic education program, explore aspects linked to their own condition.

Each chapter begins with a schematic sequence of statements together with notes as the level of scientific proof and strength of the recommendation as indicated by "Methodological Manual - How to produce, spread and update recommendations for clinical practice" drawn up under "The National Program for

Guidelines" now changed to "National System for Guidelines" (http://www.snlg-iss.it/manuale_metodologico_SNLG) (Table 1). A commentary follows, exploring the scientific basis for the proofs and the recommendations complete with bibliographical notes.

Table 1 Levels of proof and strength of the recommendation

Levels of proof
Level I: Evidence obtained from two or more properly designed randomized controlled trials
Level II: Evidence obtained from one well-designed randomized controlled trial
Level III: Evidence obtained from well-designed cohort or case-control analytic studies, preferably from more than one center or research group
Level IV: Evidence obtained from multiple time series designs with or without the intervention. Dramatic results in uncontrolled trials might also be regarded as this type of evidence
Level V: Evidence obtained by uncontrolled studies
Level VI: Opinions of respected authorities, based on clinical experience, descriptive studies, or reports of expert committees
Strength of the recommendation
Level A: Good scientific evidence suggests that performing the procedure or diagnostic test is strongly recommended
Level B: At least fair scientific evidence suggests that the benefits of the clinical service may outweigh the potential risks. Clinicians should discuss the service with eligible patients
Level C: At least fair scientific evidence suggests that there are benefits provided by the clinical service, but the balance between benefits and risks is too close for making general recommendations. Clinicians need not offer it unless there are individual considerations
Level D: The procedure or diagnostic test is not recommended
Level E: It is strongly suggested to refrain from performing the procedure or diagnostic test

Contents

Part I
General Remarks

Overview of the Management of Obese patients

1

Lucio Lucchin

1.1 Management of Obesity-Affected People

Obesity is a chronic disease with a complicated etio-pathogenesis [1, 2]. This means that the factors that make it up interact together via linear and non-linear equations, thus making the estimate of the results not precise. These factors interact and adapt themselves to the environment and culture and evolve in time. Because there is not any efficient unidirectional strategy, particularly in the long term, it is fundamental to try to give answers to questions that are not necessary in other pathologies.

1.2 Is It Strategic to Communicate Preliminarily the Typology of Treatment to the Obese Patient?

Yes, in order to limit the disorientation and the attraction towards the commercial therapeutic illusions and towards little or not competent professionals. This involves negative consequences for the obese patient, both psychologically and clinically. Doctors, *in primis*, and the other health workers who are involved in this clinical condition, have the ethical and deontological need to make their professional background transparent (especially non-doctors), besides the intervention model they are willing to adopt [3]. The Medical Deontological Italian Code (version 18 May 2014) must be considered in art. 16: diagnostic procedures and therapeutic interventions; 21: professional competence; 33: information and communication to the patient; 35: informed consensus and dissent; 55: sanitary information. The criterion

L. Lucchin
Medical Director of the Clinical Nutrition Unit Health, Distrect of Bolzano, Bolzano Hospital, Boehler street 5 39100, Bolzano, Italy
e-mail: lucio.lucchin@sabes.it

© Springer International Publishing Switzerland 2016
P. Sbraccia et al. (eds.), *Clinical Management of Overweight and Obesity: Recommendations of the Italian Society of Obesity (SIO)*,
DOI 10.1007/978-3-319-24532-4_1

of transparency of the services provided is required also at a legislative level by the Italian law 'Decreto Presidente Consiglio dei Ministri' 19 May 1995 – GU number 125: 'General reference framework of public service charter'. Even though this document is addressed to the healthcare companies, its spread is recommended to the single operative units that deal with chronic pathologies. The expectations of obese patients in terms of weight loss, which are at least 20–30 % per year [4, 5], have to be discussed ab initio. The unrealistic expectations seem not to have negative consequences [6]. In order to communicate preliminarily the treatment typology to the obese patient, it is desirable to specify:

1. Entity, organisation chart and qualifications of the operator/s
2. Way of access into the structure
3. Privacy safeguard
4. Quality standard of the unit (number of treatments per year, drop-outs after 6/12/24 months, average weight loss after 6/12/24 months, etc.)
5. Therapeutic model used with relative informed consent [7].

A preliminary meeting with everyone who has requested a reservation in a determinate time period may result useful [8]. (*Level of evidence VI, Strength of recommendation B*)

1.3   How Long Should the First and the Control Visits Last?

This aspect is underestimated, exception made for the economic aspect. In order to be efficient, the treatment of a chronical pathology needs to be clear in its contents so as to define the time needed for the medical control. In literature reports, the duration of a medical examination for an obese patient ranges between 15 and 20 min (15 min in Italian public services) [4–9]. At the present time, with an obese patient, the doctor does not modify the duration of the examinations but he modifies the contents of the examination. Most of the time is used to measure the *clinical-anthropometrical parameters* [10] and for the therapy of the complications, and just a few minutes are devoted to the finding of the strategy for changing lifestyle. The specialists in this field are used to increase the duration of the examination [11]. In order to have a good bond between efficiency and efficacy, what has to be considered to quantify the medical visit duration is:

1. Decide the minimum number of visits per year per patient (first visit + control visits).
2. Identify the components of the intervention (clinical, psychological and weight anamnesis; objective visit; patient's motivation and expectations to define targets and therapeutic strategy; prescription of the nutritional plan; etc.) and quantify their duration.
3. Plan how much information has to be given, considering that the patient remembers only a little percentage of what is said. After 30 min, the attention is at its lowest point

and 40–60 % of what the doctor said is forgotten in a couple of days. What is remembered increases to 30 % by repeating the most important concepts [12]. It is important not to give too much information all at once. Besides, it is important to remember that the patient wants to be more informed about the prognosis and about the lifestyle modification [13]; (*Kindelan and Kent in British general practice 1987*).

4. Verify the possibility of using informatics-based therapy strategies, which could be very useful and efficient if personalised and interactive [14].

In order to optimise the examination timing for the obese patient, the doctor needs to know the therapeutic education: problem solving, semantic map, empathic communication (active listening) and a good capability in understanding the non-verbal communication [1, 15, 16]. From the experience of specialists, it emerges that the average time for the first medical examination should be between 45 and 75 min, whereas the average time for a normal medical control should be between 20 and 30 min. (*Level of evidence VI, Strength of recommendation B*)

1.4   How Important Is Health Worker Example?

Health professionals should promote prevention-based strategies and encourage correct lifestyles [17]. The difficulty in becoming competent and the fact that a lot of health workers have risk factors and/or chronical pathologies that they should treat make the proposed therapeutic strategies less efficient. A part of them puts the responsibility on the patient [18], and at least one third (with growing trend) has difficulties in the proposal of adequate lifestyles due to a weak self-esteem, which is caused by the incongruence between what they do and what they suggest to the patients [19]. Literature shows how just if the doctor has a normal weight, suggest therapeutic strategies to the obese patient [20–22]. The patient as well better follows the suggestions from normal weight doctors [23]. It is also important in terms of public health that health workers are the first ones to contrast the negative stigma associated with this condition [24]. The example of the modern health worker is important for the contrast to chronicity. In order to be convincing and reassuring, it is important to improve the personal coherence level. (*Level of evidence VI, Strength of recommendation B*)

1.5   Individual or Group Therapy: Which Is the Best One?

Studies show how the individual psychological-educational intervention or the counselling one are weak in terms of efficiency as too many resources are required [25]. The group therapy (cognitive-behavioural therapy that modifies the lifestyle) seems more efficient compared to the individual treatment, especially if associated with physical activities [26]. The most favourable outcomes are related to the size of weight loss, the fat mass [27] reduction, the drop-outs, the young age, a better looking self-image [28] and a better control of food assumption after 12 months

[23]. The group therapy for the care of obesity is therefore useful, especially in public services. (*Level of evidence III, Strength of recommendation B*)

1.6 How Much Pedagogical Time Is Needed for the Obese Patient?

The complexity of obesity needs a multidimensional approach [2], based on the intervention in different fields: biological (clinical-nutritional and physical activity), psychological and socio-cultural. There are many scientific publications that state how the emotional relationship of the health worker regarding the obese patient is less than in other pathologies [29]. The loss of weight should not be considered the principal goal of the treatment of the obese patient. Weight stabilisation in a certain amount of time is linked with the pedagogical education to the pathology self-management. It has been esteemed that at the moment of the medical examination the patient has one, two–three, nine problems. The doctor finds out more or less 50 % of these problems [30]. These difficulties to identify the patients' problems are well supported in literature [31]. The perception of the consequences of overweight or obesity on the health changes from person to person but especially on the basis of the ethnic group. In order to educate the patient, it is important to improve the communication techniques that nowadays are too often inadequate [32]. The health personnel often overestimates the cognitive capacity of the patients who often say they have understood even though they have not. A patient with a chronical pathology, especially if over 65 years, has a reduced level of text comprehension (fifth level out of 12 instead of an average of eighth–ninth level) [33]. This means that the written or spoken language used has to be tested preliminarily. To remember the common learning problems: anger, denial, fright, anxiety, thoughts about health, differences of language, physical disabilities, pain, cognitive imitations, religion, age, comorbidity, economic situation, distance from the health centre. Another important factor is the therapeutic adherence that is inversely proportional to the number of pharmacological doses and to the entity of the lifestyle modification [34]. The attention to the communication methods [35] is addressed principally to language terms and style [36]. Medical practitioners are still using little systematic analysis as regards their patient's lifestyle [37]. No more than the 30 % of them motivate the patient to lose weight [38]. Scientific evidence relating to the effect of solicitation by scientific societies and/or institutions for the screening of obesity is weak [39]. An adequate counselling improves the weight loss in the long term in at least one third of the patients. The pedagogical time for the obese patient has to be esteemed in a few years and has to be included in the therapeutic strategy. The doctors who deal with obesity are recommended the implementation of:

1. Psychometric tests such as BISA (Body Image and Satisfaction Assessment), PBIA (Pictorial Body Image Assessment), HR-QoL (Health-Related Quality of Life) [40]
2. Models such as AAR (Ask, Advise and Refer) [31], FRAMES (Feedback, Responsibility, Advice, Empathy, Self-efficacy) [41] or 5A (Assess-Advise-Agree-Assist-Arrange) [9]

In the end, it results strategic to identify the various categories of obese people and, among them, the ones that could use electronic health records. (*Level of evidence III, Strength of recommendation A*)

1.7 How to Evaluate Patient Appreciation?

The detection of the treatment appreciation by the patient is fundamental in terms of quality of the service provided. The improvement of the obese patient's quality of life, which is worse than normal weight people's, is one of the primary goals of the treatment, but it should be properly supervised. The obese people are more satisfied with the treatment compared to non-obese [34]. Recently a specific survey for obesity, the Laval Questionnaire [42], has been validated. The appreciation of the treatment received and the life quality are strictly related. If there are a lot of scientific publications about the quality of life, there are not as many regarding the perceived quality of the treatment and the few existing documentations are related to the bariatric treatment [43, 44]. In this case, satisfaction has been observed from both social and physical points of view. It is recommended to predispose a systematic survey of the treatment appreciation, with adequate samples and frequency, which is fundamental for the professional improvement. (*Level of evidence V, Strength of recommendation A*)

Bibliography

1. American Medical Association & The Robert Wood Johnson Foundation, Assessment and Management of Adult Obesity: a primer for Physicians. Communication and counseling strategies. N°8 November 2003(9):1–11. www.reducingobesity.org
2. National Health Service and National Obesity Observatory (2010) Treating adult obesity through lifestyle change interventions. www.noo.org.uk/self
3. Van Genugten L, van Empelen P, Flink I, Oenema A (2010) Systematic development of a self-regulation weight-management intervention for overweight adults. BMC Public Health 27(10):649
4. Foster GD, Wadden TA, Phelan S, Sarwes DB, Sanderson RS (2001) Obese patient's perceptions of treatment outcomes and the factors that influence them. Arch Intern Med 161(24):2133–2139
5. Phelan S, Nallari M, Darroch FE, Wing RR (2009) What do physicians recommend to their overweight and obese patients? J Am Board Fam Med 22:115–122
6. Fabricatore AN, Wadden TA, Womble LG, Sarwer DB, Berkowitz RI, Foster GD, Brock JR (2007) The role of patient's expectations and goals in the behavioral and pharmacological treatment of obesity. Int J Obes 31:1739–1745
7. Lucchin L (2000) Malnutrizione: una sfida del terzo millennio per la società postindustriale. Strategia di prevenzione e cura. Il Pensiero Scientifico Editore, Rome, Exclusive vol. 617–619
8. Kob M, Schrei M, Lando L, Facchin N, D'Andrea C, Schonthaler B, Mazzoldi MA, Lucchin L (2011) Trattamento dell'obesità: l'importanza dell'accoglienza nella gestione long term della patologia cronica. ADI Mag 4:369–370
9. Schlair S, Moore S, Mc Macken M, Jay M (2012) How to deliver high-quality obesity counseling in primary care using the 5As framework. JCOM 19(5):221–229
10. Bertakis KD, Azari R (2005) The impact of obesity on primary care visit. Obes Res 13(9): 1615–1623

11. Pearson WS, Bhat-Schellbert K, Ford ES, Mokdad AH (2009) The impact of obesity on time spent with the provider and number of medications managed during office-based physician visits using a cross-sectional, national health survey. BMC Public Health 30(9):436
12. Bertakis KD (1977) The communication of information from physician to patient: a method for increasing retention and satisfaction. J Fam Pract 5:217–222
13. Kindelan K, Kent G (1986) Patients' preferences for information. J R Coll Gen Pract 36(291):461–463
14. Loucas CE, Fairburn CG, Whittington C, Pennant ME, Stockton S, Kendall T (2014) E-therapy in the treatment and prevention of eating disorders: a systematic review and meta-analysis. Behav Res Ther 63:122–131
15. WANDERSEE JH (1990) Concept mapping and the cartography of cognition. J Res Sci Teach 27(10):923–936
16. PINTO AJ, ZEITZ HJ (1997) Concept mapping: a strategy for promoting meaningful learning in medical education. Med Teach 19(2):114–120
17. Lyznicki JM, Young DC, Davis RM (2001) Council on scientific affairs, American Medical Association. Obesity: assessment and management in primary care. Am Fam Physician 63(11):2185–2196
18. Jallinoja P, Absetz P, Kuronen R, Nissinen A, Talja M, Uutela A, Patja K (2007) The dilemma of patient responsibility for lifestyle change: perceptions among primary care physicians and nurses. Scand J Prim Health Care 25(4):244–249
19. Howe M, Leidel A, Krishnan SM et al (2010) Patient related diet and exercise counseling: do providers' own lifestyle habits matter? Prev Cardiol 13:180–185. doi:10.1111/j.1751-7141.2010.00079.x
20. Bleich SN, Bennet WL, Gudzune KA, Cooper LA (2012) Impact of physician BMI on obesity care and beliefs. Obesity 20(5):999–1005
21. Puhl RM, Gold JA, Luedicke J, DePierre JA (2013) The effect of physician's body weight on patient attitudes: implications for physician selection, trust and adherence to medical advice. Int J Obesity 37:1415–1421
22. Hansra D (2014) Physicians should set an example for obese patients. Sun Sentinel 2014 april 14. www.articles.sun.sentinel.com/2014
23. Munsch S, Biedert E, Keller U (2003) Evaluation of a lifestyle change programme for the treatment of obesity in general practice. Swiss Med Wkly 133(9–10):148–154
24. Puhl RM, Hever CA (2010) Obesity stigma: important considerations for public health. Am J Public Health 100:1019–1028
25. Vila Còrocoles A, Llor Vilà C, Pellejà-Pellejà J, Gisbert Aguilar A, Jordana Ferrando P, Casacuberta Monge JM (1993) Evaluation of the effectiveness of personalized and frequent dietetic counseling in the treatment of obesity. Aten Primaria 11(6):298–300
26. Verweij LM, Coffeng J, van Mechelen W, Proper KJ (2011) Meta-analyses of workplace physical activity and dietary behaviour interventions on weight outcomes. Obes Rev 12(6):406–429
27. Renjilian DA, Perri MG, Nezu AM, McKelvey WWF, Shermer RL, Anton SD (2001) Individual versus group therapy for obesity: effects of matching participants to their treatment preferences. J Consult Clin Psychol 69(4):717–721
28. Minniti A, Bissoli L, Di Francesco V, Fantin F, Mandragona M, Olivieri M, Fontana G, Rinaldi C, Bosello O, Zamboni M (2007) Individual versus group therapy for obesity: comparison of drop-out rate and treatment out come. Eat Weight Disord 12(4):161–167
29. Gudzune KA, Beach MC, Roter DL, Cooper LA (2013) Physicians built less rapport with obese patients. Obesity 21(10):2146–2151
30. Waitzskin H (1984) Doctor-patient communication. JAMA 252:2441–2446
31. Zamosky L (2014) New obesity guidelines help physicians and patients with weight loss treatment. Med Eco 2014 february 25. www.medicaleconomics.modernmedicine.com
32. Durant NH, Barman B, Person SD, Collins F, Austin SB (2009) Patient provider communication about the health effects of obesity. Patient Educ Couns 75(1):53–57

33. Doak C, Doak LG, Root JH (1996) Teaching patients with low literacy skills, 2nd edn. JB Lippincott, Philadelphia
34. Fong RL, Bertakis KD, Franks P (2006) Association between obesity and patient satisfaction. Obesity 14:1402–1411
35. Alexander SC (2009) Ostbyealth nutrition. Session 5: nutrition communication. The challenge of effective food risk communication. Proc Nutr Soc 68(2):134–141
36. McGloin A, Delaney L, Hudson E, Wall P (2009) Symposium on the challenge of translating nutrition research into public health nutrition. Session 5: nutrition communication. The challenge of effective food risk communication. Proc Nutr Soc 68(2):134–141
37. Welborn TL, Azarian MH, Davis NJ, Layton JC, Aspy CB, Mold JW (2010) Development of an obesity counseling model based on a study of determinants of intentional sustained weight loss. J Okla State Med Assoc 103(7):243–247
38. Sonntag U, Henkel J, Renneberg B, Bockelbrink A, Braun V, Heintze C (2010) Counseling overweight patients: analysis of preventive encounter in primary care. Int J Qual Health Care 22(6):486–492
39. Smith PD, O'Halloran P, Hahn DL, Grasmick M, radant L (2010) Screening for obesity: clinical tools in evolution, a WREN study. WMJ 109(5):274–278
40. Shehab J (2013) Assessing improvement in quality of life and patient satisfaction following body contouring surgery in patients with massive weight loss: a critical review of outcomes measures employed. Plastic Surgery International. http://dx.doi.org/10.1155/2013/515737
41. Sa R, Pointer PS, Anderson JW, Noar SM, Conigliaro J (2013) Physician weight loss advice and patient weight loss behavior change: a literature review and meta-analysis of survey data. Int J Obesity 37:118–128
42. Therrien F, Marceau P, Turgeon N, Biron S, Richard D, Lacasse Y (2011) The laval questionnaire: a new instrument to measure quality of life in morbid obesity. Health Qual Life Outcomes 15(9):66
43. Dziurowicz-Kozlowska A, Lisik W, Wierzbicki Z, Kosieradzki M (2005) Health related quality of life after the surgical treatment of obesity. J Physiol Pharmacol 6:127–134
44. Pimenta GP, Saruwatari RT, Correa MR, Genaro PL, Aquilar-Nascimento JE (2010) Mortality weight loss and quality of life of patients with morbid obesity: evaluation of the surgical and medical treatment after 2 years. Arq Gastroenterol 47(3):263–269

Part II

Lifestyle Modifications

Diet Recommendations

2

Fabrizio Pasanisi, Lidia Santarpia, and Carmine Finelli

A substantial contribution to the obesity and overweight epidemic in both Western and developing countries has been given by the increase in the consumption, during growth as well as in adulthood, of foods with high energy density and low nutritional value (foods with visible fats, soft drinks with caloric sweeteners, snacks, sweets) and the strong reduction of physical activity at work and during leisure time.

The nonpharmacological treatment for overweight and obesity needs to modify unhealthy dietary habits and encourage physical activity, according to the patient's clinical conditions: in other words, a physical and nutritional rehabilitative program is often required. Moreover, an adequate integrative intervention enhances the effectiveness of the single components and optimizes the use of drugs for comorbidities; in fact, there is a well-known effective interaction between diet and physical exercise.

Treatments to correct obesity aim to reduce initial body weight – in particular for grades I and II obesity or in case of overweight – within 4–6 months. Only in case of grade III obesity it is necessary to lose more than the conventional amount of 10 %.

In substance, it has been observed that a stable loss of 10 % of the initial body weight, achieved by losing mainly fat tissue, is adequate to correct the risk of obesity-linked morbidities.

The nutritional intervention, in both public and private institutions, must never disregard a simple but thorough dietary education. When eating disorders linked with a personality disturbance are present, a psychotherapeutic clinic and diagnostic intervention is also indicated.

F. Pasanisi (✉) • L. Santarpia • C. Finelli
Department of Clinical Medicine and Surgery, Federico II University of Naples, Naples, Italy
e-mail: pasanisi@unina.it

© Springer International Publishing Switzerland 2016
P. Sbraccia et al. (eds.), *Clinical Management of Overweight and Obesity:
Recommendations of the Italian Society of Obesity (SIO)*,
DOI 10.1007/978-3-319-24532-4_2

2.1   Carbohydrates

Carbohydrates should represent 50–55 % of total calories; fiber-enriched foods and slow absorption starch should be preferred, limiting the amount of energy from simple sugars. (*Level of evidence I, Strength of recommendation A*)

Cereals, fruits, and vegetables are important components of a healthy diet and have to be taken in consideration in a regimen for obesity. (*Level of evidence I, Strength of recommendation A*)

At the moment, there is no evidence suggesting diets with low carbohydrate content (below 120–130 g/day) in obese patients. (*Level of evidence II, Strength of recommendation D*)

Simple sugars should not exceed 10–12 % of the daily energy intake; it is suggested to consume fruits and vegetables, limiting added sucrose. (*Level of evidence I, Strength of recommendation A*) [1–3]

2.2   Glycemic Index

The glycemic index of a food indicates the increase in blood glucose levels after the consumption of a food containing 50 g carbohydrates. This is influenced above all by the quality of carbohydrates (the simpler they are, the higher is the glycemic index) and by some characteristics of the meal, such as type of cooking, presence of fibers and interaction with fats and proteins.

The glycemic index needs to be considered in selecting food for the daily diet. In particular, foods with a low glycemic index have to be preferred to maintain body weight during a low-calorie diet. (*Level of evidence I, Strength of recommendation A*) [4]

2.3   Proteins

The recommended daily protein intake in adults should be 0.8–1.0 g/kg desirable weight (i.e., weight corresponding to 22.5–25 kg/m^2 BMI). Similarly, for developmental age, national nutritional recommendations should be followed. (*Level of evidence I, Strength of recommendation A*)

Proteins should derive both from animal and vegetal protein sources. (*Level of evidence I, Strength of recommendation A*) [5]

2.4   Fats

A well-balanced diet should contain less than 30 % lipids of the daily energy intake, with an optimal intake of 10 % MUFA, 10 % PUFA, 10 % saturated fatty acids. (*Level of evidence I, Strength of recommendation B*)

Daily intake of cholesterol should not exceed 300 mg/day in adults and 100 mg/1000 kcal (4190 kJ) in developmental age. (*Level of evidence I, Strength of recommendation B*)

The introduction of at least two servings of fish weekly is recommended to supply n3 polyunsaturated fatty acids, with benefits on the prevention of cardiovascular risks. (*Level of evidence II, Strength of recommendation B*)

The use of trans fatty acids has to be strongly reduced because it is associated with body weight, waist circumference, and BMI increase in population studies. It is recommended not to exceed 2.5 g/day of trans fatty acids in relation to cardiovascular risks. (*Level of evidence II, Strength of recommendation B*) [6–11]

2.5   Fiber

Dietary fiber has functional and metabolic effects. Beyond satiation and the improvement of intestinal functions, dietary fiber reduces the risk of chronic-degenerative diseases (diabetes, cardiovascular diseases) and some gastrointestinal neoplasms.

In adults, the intake of at least 30 g/day of vegetal fiber is recommended and the supplement of vegetal fibers during caloric restriction is effective to improve metabolic parameters. (*Level of evidence I, Strength of recommendation A*) [12–14]

2.6   Alcohol

Given its metabolic characteristics and the readily available calories it provides, alcohol is not recommended during a weight loss regimen since it limits the utilization of other nutrients and has no satiating power. (*Level of evidence I, Strength of recommendation B*)

Alcohol could be reintroduced in a "weight-maintenance" regimen once the patient has reached adequate weight; it should be consumed in limited doses and counted in the total daily calories prescribed [15].

2.7   Sweet Drinks

Sweetened drinks are not recommended because, as they add extra calories, they negatively influence both satiety and satiation. The patient needs to be informed about their negative effects on body weight. The consumption of sweetened drinks has to be controlled, particularly during pediatric age, because they represent a source of "empty" calories, nowadays scarcely considered by subjects with overweight/obesity and their families. (*Level of evidence I, Strength of recommendation A*) [16–18]

2.8   Sucrose and Other Added Sugars

The intake of foods containing sucrose and other added sugars should be balanced with the intake of other carbohydrates, in order to avoid exceeding the total daily calorie intake.

The excessive habitual consumption of sucrose and other added sugars could cause weight increase, insulin resistance and higher triacylglycerol blood levels. (*Level of evidence I, Strength of recommendation A*)

2.9 Special Foods, Nutritional Supplements, Noncaloric Sweeteners

Generally, there is no indication to use special foods, whether precooked or packaged. The same is true for vitamin and mineral supplements, which should be given only to patients presenting a diet history with clear nutritional deficiencies. The use of noncaloric sweeteners is controversial because they may impair both satiety and satiation.

2.10 Mediterranean Diet

The Mediterranean Diet is not correlated with an increased risk of overweight and obesity and could play a role in the prevention of both. Long-term intervention studies are required to prove the effectiveness of a Mediterranean type of diet in promoting and preventing overweight and obesity. (*Level of evidence I, Strength of recommendation B*)

The adhesion to a typical Mediterranean Diet has favorable effects on mortality for cardiovascular diseases and cancer and on the incidence of Parkinson's and Alzheimer's diseases; it therefore could play a protective role on the primary prevention of chronic-degenerative diseases. (*Level of evidence I, Strength of recommendation B*) [19–22]

2.10.1 Dietary Recommendations in Some Clinical Conditions

2.10.1.1 Diet Therapy of Obesity in Adolescence
There are no specific indications other than to empower educational programs toward healthy diet and lifestyle; regular physical exercise, and an adequate intake of proteins, minerals, and vitamins through the consumption of a large variety of natural foods, should be encouraged and stimulated.

2.10.1.2 Diet Therapy for Obesity during Pregnancy and Lactation
During pregnancy, it is sufficient to guarantee an adequate supply of proteins and foods rich in high bioavailable calcium (partially skimmed milk, yogurt, water). In particular, in the third trimester, the prescription of a diet with a caloric supply of at least 1600 kcal (6704 kJ)/day is suggested. During lactation, a woman who was overweight/obese before pregnancy could start a weight-reducing diet and try to attain a normal BMI. The energy cost for milk production is about 500–600 kcal/

day for the first 6 months of exclusive breastfeeding. For this reason and in consideration of the energy saving due to the physiological weight loss following pregnancy, national recommendations usually suggest a supply of about 500 kcal/day for a healthy woman. In overweight/obese lactating mothers, it will be sufficient to maintain a calorie supply corresponding to the real needs, without adjusting for ideal weight, since this supply will be in any case 500 kcal lower than necessary.

Particular attention is required to satisfy the increased needs in micronutrients and vitamins for milk production.

2.10.1.3 Grade III Obesity

In this case, the suggested energy intake is 1000 kcal (4190 kJ) lower than the habitual diet, with close evaluation by an expert dietitian, which includes a dietary assessment and follow-up, with special attention to pharmacological therapy of possible complications; the surgical option, in case of medical failure, has to be considered and proposed by a specialized team.

Finally, diet is a nonpharmacological therapy: it is a therapeutic intervention and has to be prescribed by physicians and elaborated by specialized personnel (dietician).

2.10.2 Specific Recommendations

Weight loss is suggested also for people with BMI between 25 and 28, in the presence of complications or personal history of diseases linked to excess body fat and in case of sarcopenia (altered fat-free/fat mass ratio): in these conditions, body weight correction has to be achieved exclusively by nonpharmacological therapy and physical rehabilitation.

Dietary restriction has to be evaluated according to the patient's energy expenditure, preferably measured (resting energy expenditure measured with indirect calorimetry in standard conditions or calculated by predictive formulas – Harris-Benedict's or WHO – and multiplied by 1.3). Generally, an energy restriction of 500–1000 kcal (2095–4190 kJ) is suggested, compared to the daily energy expenditure. Low-calorie diets with a daily caloric intake lower than 1300 kcal (5447 kJ)/day should not be prescribed to outpatients.

Diet composition should guarantee an adequate protein/nonprotein calorie ratio: the lower nonprotein calories are, the higher protein calories should be. Generally, proteins should derive from both animal and vegetal origin: 0.8–1 g proteins/kg desirable body weight is suggested (only rarely up to 1.3–1.5 g/kg desirable weight). Desirable weight corresponds to 22–25 kg/m^2 Body Mass Index calculated for the patient's squared height. As far as nonprotein calories, the amount of carbohydrates should derive from foods with low glycemic index, and fats should be of vegetal origin (limiting coconut and palm oil) and used above all for seasoning. Extra virgin olive oil should be preferred. It is advisable not to limit carbohydrate intake below 120–130 g/day and fats below 20–25 g/day.

Suggested food items are preferably vegetables, as in the Mediterranean food model: cereals, legumes, vegetables, and fruit as source of carbohydrates and a percentage of dietary proteins, lean meats, and fish (at least two–three times a week) as animal proteins, extra virgin olive oil as seasoning fat. Regular milk, yoghurt, and low-fat dairy products have to be guaranteed to ensure the protein and the calcium supply.

As to meal distribution, it is appropriate to suggest a relatively abundant breakfast (partially skimmed milk, cereals, fruits, yoghurt) and a light dinner early in the evening. A light breakfast and evening meal have no specific indications to correct obesity except for given metabolic diseases or individual requests.

2.11   Comments

Insulin resistance, with its metabolic and endocrine alterations, is commonly observed with excess body fat.

Dietary intervention (and physical rehabilitation) is aimed to counteract and decrease insulin resistance with an adequate reduction of fat mass but also to supply a well-balanced amount of macronutrients, providing a low glycemic load.

Italian dietary guidelines for healthy nutritional habits, as in all other countries with a modern national health service, are a cornerstone that should be always considered especially when representing the basics of a traditional Mediterranean diet.

Other diets, often unbalanced, i.e., diets low in carbohydrates or in lipids or with a high protein content should be considered with caution since they help reduce body weight (not necessarily body fat mass) at the beginning of the dietary intervention (usually within few weeks) but their effectiveness is poor (as far as body fat is concerned) and could be unsafe in the short as well as in the long term.

The obesity epidemic largely affects lower socioeconomic population groups; moreover, since quality foods with high nutritional value are usually more expensive than calorie dense foods with low nutritional value (the so-called empty calories) dietitians and nutrition professionals should make appropriate recommendations for adequate choices. The issue of the cost of foods for a healthy diet for everybody requires targeted national policies.

Time for cooking and food preparation should also be considered by the prescribing dietitian, as should palatability and compliance with the diet.

In summary, the cornerstones for dietary treatment of excess body fatness are:

- Always consider some physical activity according to the patient's clinical conditions.
- Prescribe a low-calorie diet with a low glycemic load.
- Achieve a 5–10 % reduction of initial body weight within four–6 months.
- Diet and physical activity are the basics for the nonpharmacological treatment of excess body fat; drugs can be added when needed.
- The prescription of diets to reduce excess body fat should consider costs and practical daily life aspects.
- Consider the vegetal fiber content of a diet.

2.12 FAQ

1. *Is diet an essential therapeutic action in the treatment of overweight/obese patients?*
   Not simply dieting but lifestyle changes should be achieved by sedentary healthy people as well as by overweight and obese patients requiring treatment.
   Treatment of obesity is not mere weight loss but the reduction of cardiovascular risk factors and the overall improvement of health status, including long-term weight loss maintenance. This can be obtained with a reasonable weight loss (about 5–10 % of initial body weight), an increasing nutritional quality of the diet, and a mild but regular physical exercise.
   Once the therapeutic target is achieved, an appropriate long-term healthy lifestyle should be observed: in other terms, the diet for obesity is part of a general program of therapeutic education.

2. *How should a diet be structured?*
   Daily food records help improve the evaluation of dietary habits and quality of foods consumed, and this tool may allow patients to recognize their feelings towards eating.
   Dietary recommendations should encourage healthy eating habits, which means including cereals, fruit and vegetables, and low-fat dairies and lean meat.
   Calorie restriction should be personalized considering the individual's social culture and traditions, taste and usual choices, habitual physical activity, comorbidities, and previous dietary programs.

3. *How should calorie restriction be carried out?*
   There is strong evidence in the literature that a diet low in fat (<30 % total calories) and a balanced intake of complex carbohydrates and proteins not only prevents weight gain in normal weight people but can also induce a modest weight loss in overweight individuals and decrease their cardiovascular risk and incidence of type 2 diabetes.
   In the short term, diets with a low glycemic load induce a body weight reduction not necessarily due to a larger loss of fat mass.
   A 15–30 % reduction of usual daily calorie intake in obese subjects with stable weight is usually adequate; frequently, patients pursue a further voluntary restriction mainly in the initial stages of the diet. It should be taken into account that energy requirements largely vary in relation to age, sex, physical activity, level of physical activity, and predisposing genetic factors, as well as previous treatments and body composition.
   A dietary regimen recommended for weight loss, targeted to individual factors, implies a reduction of 500–600 kcal/d or up to 1000 for heavy eaters. Very low calorie diets (VLCD) supplying less than 1200 kcal/d (5000 kJ/d) provide an inadequate amount of micronutrients and therefore impair the nutritional status, unfavorably affecting weight loss program. Their use is restricted to supervised patients for a short period of time. VLCD are not indicated in children, adolescents, pregnant and lactating women, or elderly obese patients.

4. *What is the right amount of macronutrients in a low-calorie diet?*
   A low-calorie diet is a nonpharmacological treatment for obese patients and should be personalized according to age, sex, excess body fat, clinical and metabolic conditions. An educational dietary program can be used for obesity prevention and weight loss maintenance. There is no standardized diet with a defined percent of macronutrient content indicating grams for kg/body weight. Daily micronutrient intake should be obtained with no less than 1200 Kcal/day, providing about 0.8–1 g protein/kg body weight, with a large variety of natural foods.

5. *What is the preferred carbohydrate and lipid intake?*
   Some studies have reported a more favorable effect on weight loss and metabolic parameters with low carbohydrate diets than with low lipid diets, although this difference is not significant in the long term, provided it is a low-calorie diet.

6. *What is the recommended protein intake?*
   An adequate protein intake should be granted during low-calorie diets. Protein intake favors satiety and maintains thermogenesis.

7. *What is the role of fibers and foods with low glycemic index in a low-calorie diet?*
   Some studies have demonstrated an increased postprandial satiety with an adequate fiber intake.

8. *How can weight regain be prevented?*
   Weight maintenance is mainly related to a physically active lifestyle. Obesity is a chronic disease and weight control is for life.

References

1. Sacks FM, Bray GA, Carey VJ et al (2009) Comparison of weight-loss diets with different compositions of fat, protein, and carbohydrates. N Engl J Med 360(9):859–873
2. Shai I, Schwarzfuchs D, Henkin Y, et al. Dietary Intervention Randomized Controlled Trial (DIRECT) Group (2008). Weight loss with a low-carbohydrate, Mediterranean, or low-fat diet. N Engl J Med. Jul 17; 359(3): 229–241
3. Surwit RS, Feinglos MN, McCaskill CC, Clay SL, Babyak MA, Brownlow BS, Plaisted CS, Lin PH (1997) Metabolic and behavioral effects of a high-sucrose diet during weight loss. Am J Clin Nutr 65(4):908–915
4. McMillan-Price J, Petocz P, Atkinson F, O'neill K, Samman S, Steinbeck K, Caterson I, Brand-Miller J (2006) Comparison of 4 diets of varying glycemic load on weight loss and cardiovascular risk reduction in overweight and obese young adults: a randomized controlled trial. Arch Intern Med 166(14):1466–1475
5. Larsen TM, Dalskov SM, van Baak M, Jebb SA, Papadaki A, Pfeiffer AF, Martinez JA, Handjieva-Darlenska T, Kunešová M, Pihlsgård M, Stender S, Holst C, Saris A, Astrup WH, Diet, Obesity, and Genes (Diogenes) Project (2010) Diets with high or low protein content and glycemic index for weight-loss maintenance. N Engl J Med 363(22):2102–2113
6. Chung H, Nettleton JA, Lemaitre RN et al (2008) Frequency and type of seafood consumed influence plasma (n-3) fatty acid concentrations. J Nutr 138(12):2422–2427
7. Foster GD, Wyatt HR, Hill JO et al (2010) Weight and metabolic outcomes after 2 years on a low-carbohydrate versus low-fat diet: a randomized trial. Ann Intern Med 153(3):147–157

8. Tapsell L, Batterham M, Huang XF, Tan SY, Teuss G, Charlton K, Oshea J, Warensjö E (2010) Short term effects of energy restriction and dietary fat sub-type on weight loss and disease risk factors. Nutr Metab Cardiovasc Dis 20(5):317–325

9. Field AE, Willett WC, Lissner L, Colditz GA (2007) Dietary fat and weight gain among women in the Nurses' health study. Obesity (Silver Spring) 15(4):967–976

10. Mozaffarian D, Katan MB, Ascherio A et al (2006) Trans fatty acids and cardiovascular disease. N Engl J Med 354:1601–1613

11. Tapsell L (2010) Short term effects of energy restriction and dietary fat sub -type on weight loss and disease risk factors. Nutr Metab Cardiovasc Dis 20:317–325

12. Maki KC, Beiseigel JM, Jonnalagadda SS, Gugger CK, Reeves MS, Farmer MV, Kaden VN, Rains TM (2010) Whole-grain ready-to-eat oat cereal, as part of a dietary program for weight loss, reduces low-density lipoprotein cholesterol in adults with overweight and obesity more than a dietary program including low-fiber control foods. J Am Diet Assoc 110(2):205–214

13. American Health Foundation (1994). Proceedings of the children's fiber conference. American Health Foundation (eds), New York

14. AAP (1993) Carbohydrates and dietary fibre. In: American Academy of Pediatrics (ed) Pediatric nutrition handbook, 3rd edn. AAD, Committee on Nutrition, Elk Grove Village

15. Colditz GA, Giovannucci E, Rimm EB, Stampfer MJ, Rosner B, Speizer FE, Gordis E, Willett WC (1991) Alcohol intake in relation to diet and obesity in women and men. Am J Clin Nutr 54(1):49–55

16. Malik VS, Schulze MB, Hu FB (2006) Intake of sugar-sweetened beverages and weight gain: a systematic review. Am J Clin Nutr 84(2):274–288

17. Vartanian LR, Schwartz MB, Brownell KD (2007) Effects of soft drink consumption on nutrition and health: a systematic review and meta-analysis. Am J Public Health 97(4):667–675

18. Chen L, Appel LJ, Loria C, Lin PH, Champagne CM, Elmer PJ, Ard JD, Mitchell D, Batch BC, Svetkey LP, Caballero B (2009) Reduction in consumption of sugar-sweetened beverages is associated with weight loss: the PREMIER trial. Am J Clin Nutr 89(5):1299–1306

19. Issa C, Darmon N, Salameh P, Maillot M, Batal M, Lairon D (2011) A Mediterranean diet pattern with low consumption of liquid sweets and refined cereals is negatively associated with adiposity in adults from rural Lebanon. Int J Obes (Lond) 35(2):251–258

20. Razquin C, Martinez JA, Martinez-Gonzalez MA, Bes-Rastrollo M, Fernández-Crehuet J, Marti A (2010) A 3-year intervention with a Mediterranean diet modified the association between the rs9939609 gene variant in FTO and body weight changes. Int J Obes (Lond) 34(2):266–272

21. Buckland G, Bach A, Serra-Majem L (2008) Obesity and the Mediterranean diet: a systematic review of observational and intervention studies. Obes Rev 9(6):582–593

22. Sofi F, Cesari F, Abbate R, Gensini GF, Casini A (2008) Adherence to Mediterranean diet and health status: meta-analysis. BMJ 337:a1344

Physical Activity

3

Pierpaolo De Feo, Emilia Sbroma Tomaro,
and Giovanni Annuzzi

3.1 Physical Activity and Global Health

More physically active people have a lower incidence of mortality by all causes, ischemic heart disease, hypertension, cerebrovascular disease, diabetes mellitus, metabolic syndrome, colon and breast cancers, and depression. They also have a better cardiorespiratory and muscle performance, a body composition, and a biochemical profile more protective for the development of cardiovascular diseases, diabetes, and bone diseases. (*Level of evidence I*)

For its positive effects on global health, regular physical activity is recommended in obese and overweight people, regardless of effects on body weight. (*Level of evidence I, Strength of recommendation A*)

In adults, at least 150 min per week of moderate-intensity aerobic physical exercise or at least 75 min of vigorous-intensity aerobic physical exercise or an equivalent combination of moderate and vigorous physical exercise are recommended, with aerobic exercise performed in periods of at least 10 min. (*Level of evidence I, Strength of recommendation A*)

To obtain further health benefits, adults can increase moderate-intensity aerobic physical exercise to 300 min per week or to 150 min of vigorous-intensity aerobic physical exercise or to an equivalent combination of moderate and vigorous aerobic physical exercise. Strength exercise, involving the main muscle groups, should be performed at least 2 days per week. (*Strength of recommendation B*)

SIO (SOCIETÀ ITALIANA DELL'OBESITÀ), Guidelines 2015.

P. De Feo (✉) • E.S. Tomaro
Healthy Lifestyle Institute CURIAMO, University of Perugia, Perugia, Italy
e-mail: pierpaolodefeo@gmail.com

G. Annuzzi
Dipartimento di Medicina Clinica e Chirurgia, University Federico II of Naples, Naples, Italy

© Springer International Publishing Switzerland 2016
P. Sbraccia et al. (eds.), *Clinical Management of Overweight and Obesity:
Recommendations of the Italian Society of Obesity (SIO)*,
DOI 10.1007/978-3-319-24532-4_3

Sedentary people will take advantage of the change from category "no activity" to "some level of activity." People who do not reach the suggested levels should increase the duration, the frequency, and at last the intensity to reach the guideline recommendations. (*Level of evidence I, Strength of recommendation A*)

3.2 Physical Activity and Prevention of Weight Gain

Regular physical activity is a protective factor for weight gain and obesity, whereas a sedentary lifestyle is a promoting factor. (*Level of evidence I*)

In adults, for prevention of a significant weight gain (more than 3 %) 150–250 min per week of moderate intensity aerobic physical exercise (corresponding to an energy expenditure of 1200–2000 kcal/5000–8400 kj) is recommended. (*Level of evidence I, Strength of recommendation A*)

3.3 Physical Activity and Treatment of Overweight and Obesity

There is a dose–response effect between the duration of physical activity and the reduction of body weight. (*Level of evidence III*). Weight loss is usually minimal with less than 150 min/week of moderate intensity aerobic physical exercise; it becomes modest with 150–250 min per week (2–3 kg in 6–12 months), whereas with 250–400 min per week it is about 5–7.5 kg in 6–12 months. (*Level of evidence II, Strength of recommendation A*)

The association between physical activity and caloric restriction significantly increases weight loss. (*Level of evidence I*)

Strength exercise, with or without caloric restriction, is not effective for weight loss. (*Level of evidence I*)

Overweight and obese people need a careful cardiorespiratory and orthopedic evaluation before and during the execution of the training program.

3.4 Physical Activity and Prevention of Weight Recovery

Physical activity levels are the best predictor of weight maintenance after a significant weight loss. (*Level of evidence I*)

At least 200 min per week of moderate intensity physical exercise is needed to prevent weight recovery. (*Level of evidence III, Strength of recommendation A*)

The more is the level of physical activity performed, the less is the weight recovery. (*Level of evidence II*)

The prescription of various types (resistance or aerobic) and doses of moderate intensity exercise training (e.g., brisk walking 135–250 min/week), delivered in the context of weight loss maintenance therapy, does not reduce the amount of weight regained after the cessation of the very low calorie diet, as compared with weight loss maintenance therapy alone. (*Level of evidence III, Strength of recommendation B*)

3.5 Comments

3.5.1 Physical Activity and Global Health

Low levels of physical activity have a strong impact on global health of populations, with a significant increase in the prevalence of noncommunicable diseases (cardiovascular diseases, diabetes, and cancer) and their risk factors (hypertension, hyperglycemia, and overweight). Considering that about the half of the disease burden in adults is currently represented by noncommunicable diseases both in industrialized and developing countries, this is a particularly relevant issue.

Sedentary lifestyle is now identified as the fourth risk factor for mortality, related to 6 % of the global deaths, after hypertension (13 %), tobacco use (9 %), and hyperglycemia (6 %), with overweight and obesity accounting for 5 % of overall mortality [1]. It is estimated that physical inactivity is the main cause of about 21–25 % of breast and colon cancers, 27 % cases of diabetes, and about 30 % cases of ischemic heart disease. According to recent estimates, elimination of physical inactivity would remove between 6 % and 10 % of the major noncommunicable diseases of CHD, type 2 diabetes, and breast and colon cancers and increase life expectancy [2, 3].

Practice of physical activity and health status are tightly linked in every age group. There is wide evidence that people with higher levels of physical activity have a lower incidence of mortality from all causes, ischemic heart disease, hypertension, cerebrovascular disease, diabetes mellitus, metabolic syndrome, colon and breast cancers, and depression [4–9]. In the EPIC study population, the hazards of all-cause mortality were 16–30 % lower in moderately inactive individuals than in those categorized as inactive in different strata of BMI and waist circumference, suggesting potential beneficial effects even with small increases in activity in inactive individuals [10]. The authors estimated that avoiding all inactivity would theoretically reduce all-cause mortality by 7.35 %, while for avoiding obesity was 3.66 % and for avoiding high waist circumference was similar to those for physical inactivity.

People who are more active also have a body composition and a biochemical profile more protective for the development of cardiovascular diseases, diabetes, and bone diseases (osteoporosis and fractures) and a better cardiorespiratory performance. Cardiorespiratory fitness (CRF) defines the ability of the circulatory, respiratory and muscular systems to supply oxygen during prolonged exercise. CRF is assessed by maximal exercise test with treadmill or cycle-ergometer and expressed as maximal uptake of oxygen (VO_2 max) or METs (metabolic equivalents, $1 MET = 3, 5$ ml O_2/kg body weight/min). CRF is a reliable marker of regular physical activity [11] and an important indicator of the health status of individuals [12]. It is associated with cardiovascular mobility and mortality, regardless of other risk factors [13–16]. A moderate or high level of CRF is associated with a lower risk of mortality from all causes in both sexes, and this protective effect is independent of age, ethnicity, adiposity, smoking habit, alcohol consumption, and health status [20, 21]. The evaluation of the dose–response relation in the meta-analysis by Kodama et al. [15], which included 33 studies with a total of 1,02,980 subjects, showed that the increase in CRF of only one MET was associated with a reduction of 13 % in mortality from all causes and 15 % in cardiovascular events. Two prospective studies that analyzed the effect of changes in CRF over time on mortality from all causes confirmed the importance of CRF as an important risk factor for mortality. Both studies, performed in males, showed that the improvement or worsening of CRF during a mean follow-up of five [22] or seven [23] years was associated with a reduction or an increase, respectively, of the mortality risk from all causes. These data support the importance of evaluating cardiorespiratory fitness in patients at cardiovascular risk and improving their CRF through training programs. A low CRF associated with a high risk of cardiovascular events was 9 MET for men and 7 MET for women in the age of 40 years, 8 and 6 MET at 50 years, and 7 and 5 MET at 60 years, respectively [15–24]. An aerobic training program in sedentary subjects can improve CRF of 1–3 MET [21] after only 3–6 months and, therefore, substantially reduce cardiovascular risk and risk of mortality from all causes.

Although the issue is still debated [27], the beneficial effects of physical activity seem to be independent of weight loss. A study evaluating the link between mortality and the degree of obesity and/or fitness showed that a low physical capacity, marker of a lower habitual physical activity, was an independent predictor of mortality from all causes, even after adjustment for adiposity; moreover, obese people with good physical capacity had a lower mortality than people of normal weight but sedentary [25].

All public health agencies and scientific organizations, such as the National Heart, Lung and Blood Institute [26] and the Centers for Disease Control in the USA, and some medical societies like the American College of Sports Medicine and the American Heart Association [27], the American Medical Association, the American Academy of Family Physicians [28] recommend regular physical activity as an important preventive and therapeutic tool also in obese and overweight people for its positive effects on global health, independently of its effect on body weight.

Although also lower amounts of physical activity showed beneficial effects on all-cause mortality in different populations [29, 30], recommendations are rather concordant in suggesting in adults at least 150 min per week of moderate-intensity aerobic physical exercise or at least 75 min of vigorous-intensity aerobic physical exercise or an equivalent combination of moderate and vigorous aerobic physical exercise. Aerobic exercise can be performed in periods of at least 10 min.

To obtain further benefits on health, adults can increase the moderate-intensity aerobic physical exercise to 300 min per week or to 150 min of vigorous-intensity physical exercise or to an equivalent combination of moderate and vigorous aerobic physical exercise.

There is limited evidence about the effectiveness of exercise against resistance in promoting the increase of or maintaining lean mass and the loss of fat mass during a low-calorie diet. However, there is evidence of favorable changes in some cardiovascular risk factors (HDL and LDL cholesterol, insulinemia, blood pressure). Strength exercise involving the main muscle groups should be performed at least 2 days per week. Maintenance of a good muscle strength reduces the risk of injuries linked to the aerobic activity.

3.5.2 Physical Activity and Prevention of Obesity

Overweight/obesity represents a multifactorial condition with complex pathophysiological interactions between genetic, endocrine, and social and environmental factors (improper dietary habits and sedentary lifestyle). There is strong scientific evidence of the protective role of an active lifestyle in the prevention of weight gain and obesity, while a sedentary lifestyle is a promoting factor [31]. Over the last decades, industrialization has brought a drastic reduction in physically active works and professions and a decreased energy consumption for transport (cars, lifts), while free time spent in nonphysically active habits (TV, computers) has considerably increased. Therefore, the modern lifestyle in developed countries, characterized by a low daily energy expenditure and a great availability of food, frequently causes a positive energetic balance with an increasing prevalence of obesity, which has become an epidemic problem of public health [32, 33].

About the prevention of weight gain, it must be stressed that primary prevention of obesity starts with the maintenance and not with the loss of weight. The risk of weight gain varies over time, and similarly it does the need to perform physical activity to prevent it. This is supported by cross-sectional evidence of an inverse relationship between weight status (weight or BMI) and physical activity [34, 35] that underlines a dose–response relation between weight loss and increasing levels of physical activity. The studies of Kavouras et al. [36] and Berk et al. [37] support the need to perform at least 150 min of physical exercise per week to control body weight for a long time. In their randomized controlled 12-month trial aiming to reach 300 min per week of moderate intensity physical exercise, McTieman et al. [38] provided further evidence about the effectiveness of more physical effort in preventing weight gain. In 5973 healthy men (mean age, 65.0 years) from the Harvard Alumni Health Study, recreational physical exercise and body weight were evaluated in 1988 (baseline), 1993, and 1998. In multivariate analyses, compared with men expending ≥ 21 MET-h per week, those expending 7.5 to <21 MET-h per week had an odds ratio (OR) of 1.35 (95 % confidence interval: 1.03, 1.77) for meaningful weight gain (≥ 3 %), and men expending <7.5 MET-h per week, an OR of 1.16 (1.01, 1.33). Therefore, those with lesser levels of physical activity were more likely to gain weight than men satisfying the 2002 IOM guidelines of ≥ 21 MET-h per week (≈ 60 min day 1 of moderate-intensity physical exercise) [39]. Very recently, the International Physical Activity and the Environment Network (IPEN) Adult study examined the dose–response associations of accelerometer-based physical activity (PA) (seven consecutive days) with BMI and weight status in 5712 adults from ten countries. Curvilinear relationships of accelerometer-based moderate-to-vigorous PA and total counts per minute with BMI and the probability of being overweight/obese were identified. The associations were negative, but weakened at higher levels of moderate to vigorous PA (450 min per day) and higher counts per minute. This was in line with current recommendations to prevent weight gain in normal-weight adults. However, complex site- and gender-specific findings for BMI were observed, which could have important implications for country-specific health guidelines [40].

These studies support the evidence that 150–250 min per week of moderate intensity physical exercise, with energetic equivalent of 1200–2000 kcal (5000–8500 kj, about 18–30 km per week), may be sufficient to prevent weight gain (>3 % of body weight) in most adults. The moderate intensity aerobic exercise should be divided into several days, with sessions lasting at least 10 min (for instance, 30 min a day for 5 days). There is no indication to strive exceeding 300 min of exercise per week, as above this threshold the benefits may not further increase while the risk of musculoskeletal injuries increases. Effective options may be performing 75 min per week of vigorous intensity aerobic physical exercise or an equivalent combination of moderate intensity and vigorous intensity exercises. Strength exercises involving the main muscle groups may be performed 2 days per week.

In line with NICE recommendations, to prevent obesity, most people may need to do 45–60 min of moderate intensity exercise a day, particularly if they do not reduce their energy intake [41].

3.5.3   Physical Activity and Weight Loss

Many studies have shown the beneficial effects of reducing weight and body fat in overweight and obese people. The use of physical activity in the therapeutic management of overweight people is essential. Weight loss is tightly linked to a negative energy balance, being a more negative energy balance associated with a greater weight loss. Since an energy deficit of 500–1000 kcal/die is necessary to reduce body weight of 0.5–1 kg per week [42], achieving this deficit only with the practice of physical activity is extremely difficult. Physical activity levels reached during military training [43] or in some sports like mountain climbing at high altitude [44] can lead to a significant weight loss; obviously obtaining and maintaining these high levels of activity is not feasible for most people. Only a few of the studies evaluating physical activity as the only mean for achieving weight loss have demonstrated a significant weight loss in overweight-obese and sedentary people, i.e., greater than or equal to 3 % of baseline weight [45]. Therefore, in the majority of obese individuals additional interventions (energy restriction or low-calorie diet) over physical activity are needed to obtain a significant weight loss [42]. A systematic review of randomized controlled trials showed that the treatment providing the most marked weight loss was the one which included physical activity, diet, and behavioral therapy [46]. The same review showed that the intensity of training should be moderate. Ross et al. [47] assessed the effectiveness of a 2-year behaviorally based physical activity and diet program implemented entirely within clinical practices. Sedentary obese adults were randomized to usual care (advice from their physicians about lifestyle as a strategy for obesity reduction) or to behavioral intervention (individual counseling from health educators to promote physical activity with a healthful diet). A significant main effect was observed for waist circumference change within the intervention compared with usual care that was sustained at 24 months for men while only at 12 months for women. The Look AHEAD trial provided evidence in patients with type 2 diabetes that weight losses achieved with intensive lifestyle intervention were still clinically meaningful (≥ 5 %) after 8-year intervention in 50 % of the participants [48].

Studies evaluating the effects of less than 150 min per week of physical exercise did not show significant weight reductions [49–52]. Donnelly et al. [53] compared the effects of 90 min per week of continuous exercise at 60–75 % of maximal aerobic capacity (30 min per session, 3 days per week), or 150 min of intermittent exercise (brisk walking, two 15-min sessions, 5 days per week), in women for 18 months. The group that performed continuous exercise lost significantly more weight (1.7 vs 0.8 kg); however, neither group lost more than 3 % of baseline weight. According to Garrow and Summerbell in a meta-analysis [54] and Wing in a review of the literature [55], the effect of physical activity on weight loss corresponded to about 2–3 kg; however, the required level of activity was not defined. In well-controlled, supervised laboratory studies it is usually evident that a greater weight loss could be related to a greater volume of activity practiced under supervision than when it is practiced independently and without supervision. In fact, Ross et al. [56] showed that males and females who underwent an energy deficit of 500–700 kcal (2095–2933 kj) in 12 weeks lost on average 7.5 kg (8 %) and 5.9 kg (6.5 %), respectively. In a randomized controlled trial of 16 months aiming at performing 225 min of moderate intensity physical exercise per week (controlled in laboratory) with energetic equivalent of 400 kcal/die (1676 kj/die), 5 days per week, Donnelly et al. [57] showed a difference between the experimental and the control group of about 4.8 kg for men and 5.2 kg for women. This result was obtained differently in the two sexes: men practicing physical activity lost weight compared to controls who kept it, whereas women practicing physical activity kept their weight compared to controls who gained it. A different response to physical activity between sexes, not confirmed in other studies [58], was also observed in the Canada's National Population Health Survey adult cohort followed over 16 years [59]. Leisure-time physical activity (LTPA) and work-related physical activity (WRPA) exerted a decreasing effect on BMI, and the effects were larger for females. Participation in LTPA exceeding 1.5 kcal/kg per day (i.e., at least 30 min of walking) reduced BMI by about 0.11–0.14 points in males and 0.20 points in females relative to physically inactive counterparts. Compared to those who were inactive at workplace, being able to stand or walk at work was associated with a reduction in BMI in the range of 0.16–0.19 points in males and 0.24–0.28 points in females. Lifting loads at workplace was associated with a reduction in BMI by 0.2–0.3 points in males and 0.3–0.4 points in females relative to those reported sedentary.

In summary, any increase in physical activity level may potentially influence weight reduction. However, based on the current evidence, activity levels <150 min per week seem not to change body weight significantly, while >150 min per week determine a modest weight loss (2–3 kg) and between 225 and 420 min cause a weight loss of 5–7.5 kg, suggesting a dose–response relationship.

Overweight and obese people need an accurate evaluation before starting a training program. Unlike the evaluation of an adult individual in good health [11], obesity needs a multidisciplinary approach, owing to its frequent comorbidities (cardiovascular, respiratory, osteoarticular). This approach should involve various professionals: internist, endocrinologist, cardiologist and specialist in sport medicine to evaluate the indications to stress test [12], orthopedic, physical therapist to evaluate the impact of the training program on the osteoarticular system. The individualized training program agreed upon by these professionals can then be managed by a graduate in physical education, preferably with master's degree in adaptive and rehabilitative sciences, with specific skills in this field.

3.5.4 Physical Activity and Maintenance of Weight Loss

Whereas the effects of physical activity alone on weight loss are minimal, physical activity has a crucial role in the management of the maintenance of body weight after weight loss. Physical activity is universally recommended to maintain body weight after having obtained a significant weight loss [4, 60], and the levels of physical activity are often considered as the best predictor of the maintenance of body weight after a significant weight loss [61, 62]. Schoeller et al. [63] showed that an expenditure of 11–12 kcal/kg/die (46.1–50.3 kj/kg/die) is necessary for an effective maintenance, whereas data from the National Weight Control Registry, including more than 3000 individuals who obtained a successful weight loss of at least 13.5 kg for a minimum of 1 year, indicate that a higher level of daily physical activity may be necessary to prevent weight recovery [64]. These individuals reported having used various methods to achieve weight loss, and more than 90 % of them emphasized the practice of high levels of physical activity as crucial for the long-term maintenance of weight.

After initial weight loss by a very low calorie diet (mean loss 13.1 kg), adding specific exercise prescriptions to the behavioral weight maintenance intervention resulted in a range of weight change at 9 months of −2.7 to +0.3 kg net of the control intervention [65]. After 33 months, participants regained weight, on average between 5.9 and 9.7 kg. The range of weight change for the exercise interventions was 3.5 to 0.2 kg less than the control weight maintenance intervention (differences not statistically significant). There were no significant differences between the two levels of recommended physical exercise—2–3 h per week of walking versus 4–6 h per week—in weight loss maintenance at 1-year postrandomization. In a study from the same group [66], after a very-low-energy diet for 2 months (mean weight loss 14.2 kg) middle-aged obese men were randomized into a walking, resistance training, or control group for 6 months while receiving similar dietary advice. At the 23-month follow-up after the weight maintenance intervention, the mean weight decrease was 4.8 kg with no statistically significant difference between the groups.

In a systematic review on this topic [67], most of the analyzed studies were observational, while in intervention studies randomization to different levels of physical activity was generally performed before weight loss and follow-up ranged from months to several years. The practice of physical activity and the recovery of weight were inversely related, and the greater the level of activity practiced the lower was the weight increase. The three studies in which randomization to physical activity occurred after having an initial weight loss showed that physical activity had a neutral, negative, or positive effect, respectively, on the prevention of weight regain.

Therefore, although physical activity may have a relevant role in the maintenance of the weight loss in obese subjects, it remains uncertain which amount is needed, also considering the interindividual variability. Although CDC/ACSM recommendations (1995) suggested to perform at least 30 min of moderate-intensity physical exercise for most of the days of the week, the long-term maintenance of weight loss seems to require performing at least 200–300 min of exercise per week. Jakicic et al. and Ewbank et al. [60, 68–71], on the basis of randomized trials, tried to define the relation between the amount of physical activity and that of maintained weight loss; in particular, they observed that the practice of at least 200 min per week of moderate intensity physical exercise determined only a minimum weight recovery after 2 years of follow-up.

Jeffery et al. [72], evaluating the effects of higher levels of physical activity (up to 2500 kcal per week; 10475 kj per week), confirmed that the higher the level of practiced activity, the lower was the weight gain.

In summary, most of the available literature on the use of physical activity for maintaining body weight after a significant weight loss suggests that "more is better." However, there are no randomized, controlled clinical trials that are specific, adequate, and of sufficient duration to allow defining the required amount.

Considering these limitations, at the present state of knowledge, weight maintenance (weight gain <3 %) can be associated to the practice of at least 60 min of walking per day at moderate intensity (about 5–6 km).

In line with NICE recommendations, the advice to people who have been obese and have lost weight is that they may need to do 60–90 min of activity a day to avoid regaining weight [41].

3.6 Definitions

Physical activity: Bodily movement produced by skeletal muscle contraction that requires an excess of energy expenditure compared to resting energy expenditure.
Physical exercise: Bodily movement that is planned, structured, repetitive and aims to improve or maintain one or more components of physical fitness.
Aerobic exercise: Rhythmic, repeated, and continuous movements of the same major muscle groups for at least 10 min each, e.g., walking, cycling, jogging, swimming, aerobic aquatic exercises.
Strength exercise: Activities that use muscular power to move a weight or work against a load offering resistance.

References

1. World Health Organization (2009) Global health risks: mortality and burden of disease attributable to selected major risks. World Health Organization, Geneva
2. American College of Cardiology/American Heart Association Task Force on Practice Guidelines, Obesity Expert Panel (2014) Expert Panel Report: Guidelines (2013) for the management of overweight and obesity in adults. Obesity (Silver Spring) 22 Suppl 2:S41–S410. doi:10.1002/oby.20660

3. Lee IM, Shiroma EJ, Lobelo F, Puska P, Katzmarzyk PT (2012) Lancet Physical Activity Series Working Group. Effect of physical inactivity on major non-communicable diseases worldwide: an analysis of burden of disease and life expectancy. Lancet 380(9838):219–229

4. Physical Activity Guidelines Advisory Committee (PAGAC) (2008) Physical activity guidelines advisory committee report. US Department of Health and Human Services, Washington, DC

5. Bauman A, Lewicka M, Schöppe S (2005) The health benefits of physical activity in developing countries. World Health Organization, Geneva

6. Warburton D et al (2007) Evidence-informed physical activity guidelines for Canadian adults. Appl Physiol Nutr Metab 32:S16–S68

7. Warburton D et al (2010) A systematic review of the evidence for Canada's Physical Activity Guidelines for Adults. Int J Behav Nutr Phys Act 7:39

8. Nocon M et al (2008) Association of physical activity with all-cause and cardiovascular mortality: a systematic review and meta-analysis. Eur J Cardiovasc Prev Rehabil 15:239–246

9. Sofi F et al (2008) Physical activity during leisure time and primary prevention of coronary heart disease: an updated meta-analysis of cohort studies. Eur J Cardiovasc Prev Rehabil 15:247–257

10. Ekelund U, Ward HA, Norat T, Luan J, May AM, Weiderpass E et al (2015) Physical activity and all-cause mortality across levels of overall and abdominal adiposity in European men and women: the European Prospective Investigation into Cancer and Nutrition Study (EPIC). Am J Clin Nutr 101(3):613–621

11. American College of Sports Medicine (1998) American College of Sports Medicine Position Stand. The recommended quantity and quality of exercise for developing and maintaining cardiorespiratory and muscular fitness, and flexibility in healthy adults. Med Sci Sports Exerc 30:975–991

12. Gibbons RJ, Balady GJ, Bricker JT, Chaitman BR, Fletcher GF, Froelicher VF et al (2002) ACC/AHA 2002 guideline update for exercise testing: summary article. A report of the American College of Cardiology/American Heart Association Task Force on Practice Guidelines (Committee to Update the 1997 Exercise Testing Guidelines). J Am Coll Cardiol 40:1531–1540

13. Carnethon MR, Gidding SS, Nehgme R, Sidney S, Jacobs DR Jr, Liu K (2003) Cardiorespiratory fitness in young adulthood and the development of cardiovascular disease risk factors. JAMA 290:3092–3100

14. Chase NL, Sui X, Lee DC, Blair SN (2009) The association of cardiorespiratory fitness and physical activity with incidence of hypertension in men. Am J Hypertens 22:417–424

15. Kodama S, Saito K, Tanaka S, Maki M, Yachi Y, Asumi M et al (2009) Cardiorespiratory fitness as a quantitative predictor of all cause mortality and cardiovascular events in healthy men and women: a meta-analysis. JAMA 301:2024–2035

16. Lee DC, Sui X, Church TS, Lee IM, Blair SN (2009) Associations of cardiorespiratory fitness and obesity with risks of impaired fasting glucose and type 2 diabetes in men. Diabetes Care 32:257–262

17. Blair SN, Kohl HW III, Paffenbarger RS Jr, Clark DG, Cooper KH, Gibbons LW (1989) Physical fitness and all-cause mortality. A prospective study of healthy men and women. JAMA 262:2395–2401

18. Gulati M, Black HR, Shaw LJ, Arnsdorf MF, Merz CN, Lauer MS et al (2005) The prognostic value of a nomogram for exercise capacity in women. N Engl J Med 353:468–475

19. Kokkinos P, Myers J, Kokkinos JP, Pittaras A, Narayan P, Manolis A et al (2008) Exercise capacity and mortality in black and white men. Circulation 117:614–622

20. Mora S, Redberg RF, Cui Y, Whiteman MK, Flaws JA, Sharrett AR et al (2003) Ability of exercise testing to predict cardiovascular and all-cause death in asymptomatic women: a 20-year 34 journal of psychopharmacology 24(11) follow-up of the lipid research clinics prevalence study. JAMA 290:1600–1607

21. Sandvik L, Eriksson J, Thaulow E, Eriksen G, Mundal R, Rodahl K (1993) Physical fitness as a predictor of mortality among healthy, middle-aged Norwegian men. N Engl J Med 328:533–537

22. Erikssen G, Liestol K, Bjornholt J, Thaulow E, Sandvik L, Erikssen J (1998) Changes in physical fitness and changes in mortality. Lancet 352:759–762

23. Blair SN, Kohl HW III, Barlow CE, Paffenbarger RS Jr, Gibbons LW, Macera CA (1995) Changes in physical fitness and all cause mortality. A prospective study of healthy and unhealthy men. JAMA 273:1093–1098
24. Fogelholm M (2010) Physical activity, fitness and fatness: relations to mortality, morbidity and disease risk factors. A systematic review. Obes Rev 11:202–221
25. Sui X, LaMonte MJ, Laditka JN et al (2007) Cardiorespiratory fitness and adiposity as mortality predictors in older adults. JAMA 298:2507–2516
26. Expert Panel on the Identification, Evaluation, and Treatment of Overweight in Adults. Clinical guidelines on the identification, evaluation, and treatment of overweight and obesity in adults: executive summary (1–3). Am J Clin Nutr. 1998;68:899–917
27. Haskell WL, Lee IM, Pate RR et al (2007) Physical activity and public health: updated recommendation for adults from the American College of Sports Medicine and the American Heart Association. Med Sci Sports Exerc 39(8):1423–1434
28. Lyznicki JM, Young DC, Riggs JA, Davis RM (2001) Obesity: assessment and management in primary care. Am Fam Physician 63:2185–2196
29. Wen CP, Wai JP, Tsai MK, Yang YC, Cheng TY, Lee MC, Chan HT, Tsao CK, Tsai SP, Wu X (2011) Minimum amount of physical activity for reduced mortality and extended life expectancy: a prospective cohort study. Lancet 378(9798):1244–1253
30. Arem H, Moore SC, Patel A, Hartge P, de Berrington GA, Visvanathan K, Campbell PT, Freedman M, Weiderpass E, Adami HO, Linet MS, Lee IM, Matthews CE (2015) Leisure time physical activity and mortality: a detailed pooled analysis of the dose–response relationship. JAMA Intern Med 175(6):959–967
31. Joint FAO/WHO Expert Consultation (2003) Diet, nutrition and the prevention of chronic diseases, vol 916, WHO technical report series. World Health Organization, Geneva
32. Brock DW, Thomas O, Cowan CD, Allison DB, Gaesser GA, Hunter GR (2009) Association between insufficiently physically active and the prevalence of obesity in the United States. J Phys Act Health 6:1–5
33. Baba R, Iwao N, Koketsu M, Nagashima M, Inasaka H (2006) Risk of obesity enhanced by poor physical activity in high school students. Pediatr Int 48:268–273
34. Ball K, Owen N, Salmon J, Bauman A, Gore CJ (2001) Associations of physical activity with body weight and fat in men and women. Int J Obes Relat Metab Disord 25:914–919
35. Martinez JA, Kearney JM, Kafatos A, Paquet S, Martinez-Gonzalez MA (1999) Variables independently associated with self reported obesity in the European Union. Public Health Nutr 2:125–133
36. Kavouras SA, Panagiotakos DB, Pitsavos C et al (2007) Physical activity, obesity status, and glycemic control: the ATTICA study. Med Sci Sports Exerc 39(4):606–611
37. Berk DR, Hubert HB, Fries JF (2006) Associations of changes in exercise level with subsequent disability among seniors: a 16-year longitudinal study. J Gerontol A Biol Sci Med Sci 61(1):97–102
38. McTiernan A, Sorensen B, Irwin ML et al (2007) Exercise effect on weight and body fat in men and women. Obesity 15:1496–1512
39. Shiroma EJ, Sesso HD, Lee IM (2012) Physical activity and weight gain prevention in older men. Int J Obes (Lond) 36(9):1165–1169
40. Van Dyck D, Cerin E, De Bourdeaudhuij I, Hinckson E, Reis RS, Davey R et al (2015) International study of objectively measured physical activity and sedentary time with body mass index and obesity: IPEN adult study. Int J Obes (Lond) 39(2):199–207
41. Stegenga H, Haines A, Jones K, Wilding J (2014) Guideline Development Group. Identification, assessment, and management of overweight and obesity: summary of updated NICE guidance. BMJ 349:g6608
42. Adult weight management evidence-based nutrition practice guideline. American Dietetic Association evidence analysis library. Web site. http://www.adaevidencelibrary.com/topic.cfm?cat=2798
43. Nindl BC, Barnes BR, Alemany JA, Frykman PN, Shippee RL, Friedl KE (2007) Physiological consequences of U.S. Army Ranger training. Med Sci Sports Exerc 39(8):1380–1387
44. Pulfrey SM, Jones PJ (1996) Energy expenditure and requirement while climbing above 6,000 m. J Appl Physiol 81:1306–1311

34

P. De Feo et al.

45. Physical activity and health: a report of the Surgeon General. Centers for Disease control and Prevention. Web site. http://www.cdc.gov/nccdphp/sgr/contents.htm
46. Södlerlund A, Fischer A, Johansson T (2009) Physical activity, diet and behaviour modification in the treatment of overweight and obese adults: a systematic review. Perspect Public Health 129(3):132–142
47. Ross R, Lam M, Blair SN, Church TS, Godwin M, Hotz SB, Johnson A, Katzmarzyk PT, Lévesque L, MacDonald S (2012) Trial of prevention and reduction of obesity through active living in clinical settings: a randomized controlled trial. Arch Intern Med 172(5):414–424
48. Look AHEAD Research Group (2014) Eight-year weight losses with an intensive lifestyle intervention: the look AHEAD study. Obesity (Silver Spring) 22(1):5–13
49. Boudou P, Sobngwi E, Mauvais-Jarvis F, Vexiau P, Gautier JF (2003) Absence of exercise-induced variations in adiponectin levels despite decreased abdominal adiposity and improved insulin sensitivity in type 2 diabetic men. Eur J Endocrinol 149:421–424
50. Campbell KL, Westerlind KC, Harber VJ, Bell GJ, Mackey JR, Courneya KS (2007) Effects of aerobic exercise training on estrogen metabolism in premenopausal women: a randomized controlled trial. Cancer Epidemiol Biomarkers Prev 16:731–739
51. Dengel DR, Galecki AT, Hagberg JM, Pratley RE (1998) The independent and combined effects of weight loss and aerobic exercise on blood pressure and oral glucose tolerance in older men. Am J Hypertens 11:1405–1412
52. Murphy M, Nevill A, Biddle S, Neville C, Hardman A (2002) Accumulation brisk walking for fitness, cardiovascular risk, and psychological health. Med Sci Sports Exerc 34(9):1468–1474
53. Donnelly JE, Jacobsen DJ, Snyder Heelan KA, Seip R, Smith S (2000) The effects of 18 months of intermittent vs continuous exercise on aerobic capacity, body weight and composition, and metabolic fitness in previously sedentary, moderately obese females. Int J Obes Relat Metab Disord 24:566–572
54. Garrow JS, Summerbell CD (1995) Meta-analysis: effect of exercise, with or without dieting, on the body composition of overweight subjects. Eur J Clin Nutr 49:1–10
55. Wing R (1999) Physical activity in the treatment of the adulthood overweight and obesity: current evidence and research issues. Med Sci Sports Exerc 31:S547–S552
56. Ross R, Pedwell H, Rissanen J (1995) Effects of energy restriction and exercise on skeletal muscle and adipose tissue in women as measured by magnetic resonance imaging. Am J Clin Nutr 61:1179–1185
57. Donnelly JE, Pronk NP, Jacobsen DJ, Pronk SJ, Jakicic JM (1991) Effects of a very-low-calorie diet and physical-training regimens on body composition and resting metabolic rate in obese females. Am J Clin Nutr 54:56–61
58. Stefanick ML, Mackey S, Sheehan M, Ellsworth N, Haskell WL, Wood PD (1998) Effects of diet and exercise in men and postmenopausal women with low levels of HDL cholesterol and high levels of LDL cholesterol. N Engl J Med 339:12–20
59. Sarma S, Zaric GS, Campbell MK, Gilliland J (2014) The effect of physical activity on adult obesity: evidence from the Canadian NPHS panel. Econ Hum Biol 14:1–21
60. Jakicic JM, Clark K, Coleman E et al (2001) Appropriate intervention strategies for weight loss and prevention of weight regain for adults. Med Sci Sports Exerc 33(12):2145–2156
61. Klem ML, Wing RR, McGuire MT, Seagle HM, Hill JO (1997) A descriptive study of individuals successful at long-term maintenance of substantial weight loss. Am J Clin Nutr 66:239–246
62. Tate DF, Jeffery RW, Sherwood NE, Wing RR (2007) Long-term weight losses associated with prescription of higher physical activity goals. Are higher levels of physical activity protective against weight regain? Am J Clin Nutr 85:954–959
63. Schoeller DA, Shay K, Kushner RF (1997) How much physical activity is needed to minimize weight gain in previously obese women? Am J Clin Nutr 66:551
64. Catenacci VA, Ogden LG, Stuht J, Phelan S, Wing RR, Hill JO, Wyatt HR (2008) Physical activity patterns in the National Weight Control Registry. Obesity 16:153–161
65. Fogelholm M, Kukkonen-Harjula K, Nenonen A, Pasanen M (2000) Effects of walking training on weight maintenance after a very-low-energy diet in premenopausal obese women: a randomized controlled trial. Arch Intern Med 160(14):2177–2184

66. Kukkonen-Harjula KT, Borg PT, Nenonen AM, Fogelholm MG (2005) Effects of a weight maintenance program with or without exercise on the metabolic syndrome: a randomized trial in obese men. Prev Med 41(3–4):784–790
67. Fogelholm M, Kukkonen-Harjula K (2000) Does physical activity prevent weight gain-a systematic review. Obes Rev 1:95–111
68. Jakicic JM, Marcus BH, Gallagher KL, Napolitano M, Lang W (2003) Effect of exercise duration and intensity on weight loss in overweight, sedentary women. JAMA 290:1323
69. Jakicic JM, Marcus BH, Lang W, Janney C (2008) Effect of exercise on 24-month weight loss maintenance in overweight women. Arch Intern Med 168:1550–1559; discussion 1559–1560
70. Jakicic JM, Winters C, Lang W, Wing RR (1999) Effects of intermittent exercise and use of home exercise equipment on adherence, weight loss, and fitness in overweight women. JAMA 282(16):1554–1560
71. Ewbank PP, Darga LL, Lucas CP (1995) Physical activity as a predictor of weight maintenance in previously obese subjects. Obes Res 3(3):257–263
72. Jeffery RW, Wing RR, Sherwood NE, Tate DF (2003) Physical activity and weight loss: does prescribing higher physical activity goals improve outcome? Am J Clin Nutr 78:684–689

Therapeutic Education

4

Carlo Rotella, Barbara Cresci, Laura Pala, and Ilaria Dicembrini

> Therapeutic Education means the therapeutic act continuously characterized by "accompanying" the patient, "joining together" in the path of chronic disease, tending to negotiate, agree, for the implementation of measures aimed at achieving the highest possible clinical outcome and the best perceived quality of life for each patient.
>
> Valerio Miselli

Therapeutic education, as defined by the WHO in 1998, should allow the patients to acquire and maintain the skills that allow them to achieve the optimal management of their lives with the disease. Its importance is recognized for the first time in 1972 by the work of L. Miller [1], which becomes a continuous process integrated in health care. Therapeutic education is an essential part in the management of chronic patients. Its purpose is to implement the knowledge about the disease and its management and to change the associated behaviors in order to achieve a better management of the disease itself. Moreover, education allows us to understand and

> **Recommendations and Grades of Evidence**
> The techniques of behavioral therapy, in addition to lifestyle modification, are more effective in the treatment of obese patients compared to intervention on lifestyle only. (*Level of evidence I, Strength of recommendation A*)
>
> Therapeutic education for the short-medium term obesity is most effective when planned and organized for small groups of patients. (*Level of evidence I, Strength of recommendation A*)

C. Rotella (✉)
Dipartimento di Scienze Biomediche, Sperimentali e Cliniche "Mario Serio",
Università di Firenze, Florence, Italy
e-mail: c.rotella@dfc.unifi.it

B. Cresci • L. Pala • I. Dicembrini
Azienda Ospedaliera Universitaria Careggi, Sod Diabetologia,
University of Florence, Florence, Italy

© Springer International Publishing Switzerland 2016
P. Sbraccia et al. (eds.), *Clinical Management of Overweight and Obesity: Recommendations of the Italian Society of Obesity (SIO)*,
DOI 10.1007/978-3-319-24532-4_4

Therapeutic education of obesity should be guaranteed, within the team, by professionals (doctor, nurse, dietitian, community health educator) specifically qualified on the basis of a continuing training on educational activities. (*Level of evidence I, Strength of recommendation A*)

Motivation is crucial to achieve therapeutic adherence and weight loss. (*Level of evidence I, Strength of recommendation A*)

Table 4.1 Cornerstones of Therapeutic Education

Among the techniques derived from cognitive behavioral therapy that represent the cornerstones of therapeutic education, we find the following ones:
1. Therapeutic alliance
2. Therapeutic adherence
3. Motivation
4. Problem solving
5. Empowerment
6. Narrative medicine

manage the psychological aspects related to the disease and therefore, in addition to the role of information on the practical management of the disease, it aims at improving the quality of life [2–6] (Table 4.1).

4.1 The Therapeutic Alliance

The continuous management of the patient affected by a chronic disease has to be evaluated in a time perspective because it is the main core of the therapeutic contract. The therapeutic contract needs to actively involve both the patient and the therapeutic team. The aims of this relationship, according to the clinical setting, have to be carefully discussed and defined. The therapeutic alliance, as a sort of deal, is able to improve, both on the short and the long term, the outcomes of the clinical management of patients affected by a chronic disease. Supporting patients makes them feel motivated and ready to change lifestyle and to actively follow the therapy. A prescriptive approach coming from health care professionals has to be left behind today. The subject affected by a chronic disease cannot be considered as a passive receptacle; he needs to be recognized as the main character of the therapeutic alliance [7–9].

4.2 The Therapeutic Adherence

The therapeutic aims of the clinical management of chronic diseases require, first of all, behavioral changes to improve lifestyle and adherence to the drug treatment. Patients affected by a chronic disease can reach the therapeutic goals only if they get to feel them of great importance for their own health status. For this reason, the term of compliance has been widely introduced in the clinical practice. The compliance has to be considered as the adherence of the patient to the therapeutic scheme. This aspect can often generate some concerns between patient and health care professionals: the therapeutic relationship usually becomes an act of force, then the patient feels to be abducted by the external pressure, warning, and intimidation coming from health care professionals. For this reason, the therapeutic adherence has been changed across the time in therapeutic adherence, thus to underline the need for an active involvement of the patient in the therapeutic decision [10–12].

4.3   Motivation

Weight management programs still remain a great challenge as drop-out rates represent a growing problem. It is essential to try and identify the predictors of success in order to make a proposal really custom-tailored to the patients. Among the most valuable applications of valid weight loss prediction models is the early identification of individuals with the least estimated probability of success, who should be directed to alternative therapies. Equally important are improvements in the matching between treatments and participants, which are dependent on the measurement of relevant pretreatment variables. In the treatment of obesity and in many other pathologies and dependencies, the motivation to change plays an important role both in the period of the weight loss and in the phase of the maintenance of the result [13]. The meaning of motivation can be variously indicated as:

- The needs, the beliefs that determine a character
- The push to carry out an action
- The tendency to devote energies to achieve a goal
- Feelings leading an individual towards a particular object

   The term motivation comes from the Latin *motus*, literally the "push of a subject towards an object," which well expresses the importance of such a predisposition for the achievement of a stable change in lifestyle, as an objective of therapeutic education. Specifically, what determines a real push for change is the presence of what is called motivational readiness, a concept that implies the existence of a real push towards the goal but in the presence of a state of readiness, which is a current and effective willingness to start the treatment. A person may believe to be motivated without really being motivated. In this case, the conflict that is present in the starting condition (for example, the status of obesity) actually prevents the patient to easily move away from that condition. A subject may also be motivated without being ready, because there are serious obstacles that prevent him from facing the problem.
   The motivation to change can go through these different stages several times before a stable change is finally reached. The stages of change are represented by the meditation (the subject is aware of the problem, sometimes accepts the change, sometimes rejects it), the determination (phase limited in time during which the decision to change may occur), the action (beginning of the change), the maintaining (with an active work of consolidation and relapse prevention), and finally the fallout (if you are not completely out of the problem, a relapse may occur) [14].

The motivation to change must therefore preexist in the patient as a substrate of his therapeutic path, but at the same time the clinician has the task of directing it towards the proposed educational project in order to ensure the therapeutic alliance with the patient. Equally important for the clinician it is also to know how to reinforce the motivational readiness in the patient during the different phases of the treatment, in order to improve the adherence and the implementation of the care project [13, 15]. Therefore, if the patient is considered to be ready to lose weight, weight loss therapy should be initiated, if not the immediate goal should be to prevent further weight gain and to try and identify the obstacles to weight reduction. In a few words, candidates for treatment are patients who decide they want to lose weight for appropriate reasons, are not currently experiencing major life stress factors, do not have psychiatric or medical illnesses that prevent effective weight loss, and are willing to devote the necessary time to make lifestyle changes.

4.4 Problem Solving

Problem solving consists in one of the most widely used method in medicine for making the patient able to usefully change his behavior. The right management of external stimuli, thoughts, and emotions is of critical importance to overcome the loss of their usual habits concerning diet and physical exercise. Problem solving is a method of self-analysis which can make the patient able to improve the relationship with food, significantly decreasing the loss of control on food intake. Through this approach, the patient can develop self-analysis skills to promptly identify hazardous situations and subsequently appropriately manage his own dietary habits and lifestyle. This strategy has different steps: the first one regarding the acknowledgment of hazardous situations or "the hurdle," the following ones focusing on the different solution paths which can be evaluated and executed, and at last on the identification of the best possible solution to carry out [16–18].

4.5 Empowerment

The literal definition of empowerment would be "empowerment" or rather "the set of knowledge, skills and relational skills that allow an individual or a group to set goals and develop strategies to achieve them by using existing resources." Empowerment is a process of social action through which individuals, organizations, and communities acquire jurisdiction over their lives, in order to change their social and political environment to improve equity and quality of life. From this, it emerges that empowerment is both a concept and a process that allows you to reach the goals. Two are the main drivers of empowerment: the feeling of being able to make effective action to achieve a goal and the ability to perceive the influence of one's actions on events. In this sense it emerges the importance of the search for a sense of confidence and self-efficacy by which the individual will be encouraged to "learn to do" and then to "do." The patient becomes conscious of being effective in changing the events of his life, in implementing his self-esteem, and in interpreting failures as learning moments.

On the basis of these assumptions, even the role of the physician changes, becoming a figure who accompanies the patient to share his decisions, stimulates his autonomy and his sense of responsibility, identifies his needs, and promotes his personal growth [1, 19].

Besides the figure of the physician, also the empowerment of the patient's family can be advisable, especially as regards the approach to childhood obesity, which can become an added value in achieving the therapeutic goal [20].

4.6 Narrative Medicine

Narrative medicine uses autobiography as an instrument through which a patient with a chronic disease may find new strategies and energy to face his own life. The goal is to make the patient write a biography of his disease in order to stimulate him to take care of himself and his disease. As a matter of fact, a greater awareness of his own history does change the way the patient looks at his present and future, stimulating new ideas and new ways of interpretation. In addition, this instrument stimulates the patient's self-care and responsibility by strengthening already existing resources [21].

In everyday life, we use our narrative ability to tell ourselves to others, to say something about us, about our past and also about our future expectations. Similarly, the patient tells the doctor his "history of the disease," and this is the truest and most complete description of his malaise. GG Marquez says: "Life is not what you experience but what you remember and how you remember to tell it."

Narrative medicine, among whose founders there are two Harvard psychiatrists, Kleinman and Good, thus deserves the attention it is receiving in recent times. Today, at a time when medicine has reached extraordinary achievements in technological development and the concept of evidence-based medicine is very familiar, the need has been felt to recover a doctor-patient relationship where the narrative of the patient's pathology to the doctor is considered like the clinical signs and symptoms of the disease itself. This narrative medicine (NBM, narrative-based medicine) refers not only to the patient's experience but also to the experiences of the doctor-patient relationship. Recently a new model of care based on narrative medicine has been developed. This new model allows an accurate assessment of the decision-making ability without the ethical and philosophical problems present in the traditional model. Further studies could explore the reliability of evaluation capacity with the narrative model [22].

References

1. Miller LV, Goldstein J (1972) More efficient care of diabetic patients in a country-hospital setting. N Engl J Med 286:1388–1391
2. Rotella CM (2005) Il ruolo dell'Educazione terapeutica nel trattamento dell'obesità e del diabete mellito. SEE, Firenze
3. Shaw KA, O'Rourke P, Del Mar C, Kenardy J (2005) Psychological Interventions for overweight or obesity. Cochrane Database. Art No: CD003818. doi:10.1002/14651858.CD003818. pub2

4. Stubbs J, Whybrow S, Teixeira P, Blundell J, Lawton C, Westenhoefer J, Engel D, Shepherd R, Mcconnon Á, Gilbert P, Raats M (2011) Problems in identifying predictors and correlates of weight loss and maintenance: implications for weight control therapies based on behaviour change. Obes Rev 12(9):688–708

5. Cresci B, Tesi F, La Ferlita T, Ricca V, Ravaldi C, Rotella CM, Mannucci E (2007) Group versus individual cognitive-behavioral treatment for obesity: results after 36 months. Eat Weight Disord 12(4):147–153

6. Briançon S, Bonsergent E, Agrinier N, Tessier S, Legrand K, Lecomte E, Aptel E, Hercberg S, Collin JF, PRALIMAP Trial Group (2010) PRALIMAP: study protocol for a high school-based, factorial cluster randomized interventional trial of three overweight and obesity prevention strategies. Trials 11:119

7. Allison DB, Elobeid MA, Cope MB, Brock DW, Faith MS, Vander Veur S, Berkowitz R, Cutter G, McVie T, Gadde KM, Foster GD (2010) Sample size in obesity trials: patient perspective versus current practice. Med Decis Making 30(1):68–75

8. Prochaska J, Di Clemente C (1986) Towards a comprehensive model of change. In: Miller W, Heather N (eds) Treating addictive behaviours: process of change. Plenum Press, New York, pp 3–27

9. Fuertes JN, Mislowack A, Bennett J, Paul L, Gilbert TC, Fontan G, Boylan LS (2007) The physician-patient working alliance. Patient Educ Couns 66(1):29–36

10. Kreps GL, Villagran MM, Zhao X, McHorney CA, Ledford C, Weathers M, Keefe B (2011) Development and validation of motivational messages to improve prescription medication adherence for patients with chronic health problems. Patient Educ Couns 83(3):375–381

11. Doggrell SA (2010) Adherence to medicines in the older-aged with chronic conditions: does intervention by an allied health professional help? Drugs Aging 27(3):239–254

12. Deccache A, van Ballekom K (2010) From patient compliance to empowerment and consumer's choice: evolution or regression? an overview of patient education in French speaking European countries. Patient Educ Couns 78(3):282–287

13. Cresci B, Rotella CM (2009) Motivational readiness to change in lifestyle modification programs. Eat Weight Disord 14(2–3):e158–e162

14. Prochaska JO, Di Clemente CC (1983) Stages and processes of self-change of smoking: toward an integrative model of change. J Consult Clin Psychol 51:390–395

15. Cresci B, Castellini G, Pala L, Ravaldi C, Faravelli C, Rotella CM, Ricca V (2011) Motivational readiness for treatment in weight control programs: the TREatment MOtivation and REadiness (TRE-MORE) test. J Endocrinol Invest 34(3):e70–e77

16. Keskin G, Engin E, Dulgerler S (2010) Eating attitude in the obese patients: the evaluation in terms of relational factors. J Psychiatr Ment Health Nurs 17(10):900–908

17. Crépin C, Carrard I, Perroud A, Van der Linden M, Golay A (2010) Managing impulsivity in obesity with problem solving. Rev Med Suisse 6(231):46–50

18. Foreyt JP (2006) The role of lifestyle modification in dysmetabolic syndrome management. Nestle Nutr Workshop Ser Clin Perform Programme 11:197–205

19. Wilson N, Minkler M, Dasho S, Wallerstein N, Martin AC (2008) Getting to social action: the Youth Empowerment Strategies (YES!) project. Health Promot Pract 9(4):395–403, Epub 2006 Jun 27

20. Jurkowski JM, Lawson HA, Green Mills LL, Wilner PG 3rd, Davison KK (2014) The empowerment of low-income parents engaged in a childhood obesity intervention. Fam Community Health 37(2):104–118

21. Maldonato A, Piana N, Bloise D, Baldelli A (2010) Optimizing patient education for people with obesity: possible use of the autobiographical approach. Patient Educ Couns 79(3):287–290, Epub 2010 Mar 29

22. Mahr G (2015) Narrative medicine and decision making capacity. J Eval Clin Pract 21(3):503–507

Part III

Treatment

Pharmacological Management

5

Enzo Nisoli and Fabrizio Muratori

Over the past 25 years, more than 120 drugs have been studied for the treatment of obesity. Orlistat is the only drug approved in the United States and Italy for the long-term therapy. The other drugs studied for a long-term treatment, sibutramine[1] and rimonabant, were withdrawn from market for safety problems [1, 2].

5.1 General Information and Therapy Initiation

In Italy the anti-obesity drug therapy is restricted to adults, while in the United States, orlistat use is allowed in patients over 12 years of age.

5.1.1 Adult Patients

Drug therapy should be considered only after effectiveness of diet and exercise and, where recommended, cognitive behavioral therapy has been assessed, and these therapeutic approaches have proved to be ineffective either to induce weight loss or to maintain weight loss. (*Level of Evidence II, Strength of Recommendation B*)

---

[1] Sibutramine was withdrawn in Europe by EMA in January 2010, after SCOUT study showing a higher number of nonfatal cardiovascular and cerebrovascular events in patients affected by cardiovascular disease and diabetes and, thus, contraindicated for the use of this drug.

E. Nisoli (✉)
Department of Biomedical Technology and Translational Medicine,
University of Milan, Milan, Italy
e-mail: enzo.nisoli@unimi.it

F. Muratori
Unit of Endocrinology, Diabetology and Clinical Nutrition, Como Hospital,
Como, Italy

© Springer International Publishing Switzerland 2016
P. Sbraccia et al. (eds.), *Clinical Management of Overweight and Obesity: Recommendations of the Italian Society of Obesity (SIO)*,
DOI 10.1007/978-3-319-24532-4_5

When it is possible, the decision on whether to start a drug therapy and what drug to choose should be made after discussion with the patient on the benefits and potential limitations of the drug, including its mechanism of action, side effects, and possible impact on motivation to lose weight. When prescribing drug therapy, the practitioner should provide information, support and counseling on diet, physical activity, and behavioral strategies to be adopted. (*Level of Evidence I, Strength of Recommendation A*)

5.1.2   Pediatric Patients

Drug treatment is not generally recommended for children under 12 years of age. As already mentioned, in the United States, unlike Italy, the use of orlistat has been authorized in children older than 12 years. (*Level of Evidence II, Strength of Recommendation B*)

5.1.2.1 Continuation of Therapy and Discontinuation of the Drug
Drug treatment may be suggested in order to maintain the weight loss rather than to induce further weight loss. The suggestion of cyclic or intermittent therapy has been reached in this context of thoughts.[2] (*Level of Evidence II, Strength of Recommendation C*)

When there are concerns about the adequate intake of micronutrients, the practitioner should take into consideration the opportunity to supplement patient with dietary vitamins and minerals, particularly with the most vulnerable groups of patients, such as the elderly (itself at risk of malnutrition) and young people (that need vitamins and minerals for the growth and development). (*Level of Evidence II, Strength of Recommendation C*)

We recommend to check regularly the anti-obesity treatment to monitor the effects of the drugs and to reinforce nutritional advice and adherence to healthy lifestyles. (*Level of Evidence I, Strength of Recommendation A*)

The suspension of drug treatment should be considered in patients who do not lose body weight. (*Level of Evidence II, Strength of Recommendation C*)

The speed of weight loss may be slower in patients with type 2 diabetes. (*Level of Evidence I, Strength of Recommendation A*). Thus, the goals of therapy may be less stringent in these than nondiabetic patients.

These goals should be agreed with the patient and reassessed regularly during treatment. At drug suspension, the patients should be supported adequately to maintain the weight loss. (*Level of Evidence I, Strength of Recommendation A*)

---

[2] A relevant question with drug therapy is to decide whether such therapy must be continuous or intermittent. In the few studies undertaken to clarify this matter and conducted according to the criteria required by the FDA, the intermittent therapy has found to provide results substantially comparable to the long-lasting therapy.

5.2   Orlistat

Orlistat should be administered only as one of the diverse treatment tools in a comprehensive, anti-obesity treatment plan to adult patients who meet the following
criteria:

- $BMI \geq 27.0$ kg/m^2 with associated risk factors
- $BMI \geq 30.0$ kg/m^2

Therapy should be prolonged beyond 3 months only if patients have lost ~5 %
body weight from the starting time of drug therapy. (*Level of Evidence II, Strength
of Recommendation C*)

The decision to use the drug for more than 24 months (usually for weight maintenance) should be made after careful discussion with the patient about potential
side effects and limits of the drug treatment. (*Level of Evidence II, Strength of
Recommendation C*)

5.3   Comments

Overall, the efficacy of anti-obesity drugs is considered to be modest, with placebo-
subtracted weight loss of <5 kg after 1 year of treatment with either orlistat,
rimonabant, or sibutramine [3]. Although apparently modest, this result is relevant
in clinics because the drug effect significantly increases the number of patients who
obtain a decrease of body weight higher than 5–10 % as compared to the initial
weight after 1 year of therapy [4]. Discontinuation of pharmacotherapy, as well as
the interruption of the other therapeutic approaches, is accompanied by recovery of
the lost weight [4]. Combination therapy with two oral agents (orlistat and sibutramine) did not prove to be superior to single-agent therapy [3]. Nevertheless, the
association of two active substances is the conceptual basis of new drugs in advanced
study phase (see below).

It is important to stress that the anti-obesity drugs should not be considered only
as a therapy to reduce weight but rather as therapeutic tools that permit weight management and thus facilitate weight maintenance over time. Moreover, drug therapy
is able to improve the metabolic profile of obese patients suffering of obesity-related
diseases. Finally, the use of drugs in obesity therapy must be considered as a help in
facilitating the adherence of patients to treatment, which also does include lifestyle
changes (i.e., diet and exercise) and cognitive behavioral therapy. Drug therapy
should be considered in patients with a $BMI \geq 30$ kg/m^2 unresponsive to diet and
exercise or with a $BMI > 27$ kg/m^2 with obesity-related complications.[3] Once an
anti-obesity drug is prescribed, patients should be actively engaged in a program of
lifestyle intervention providing strategies and tools needed to achieve significant
weight loss and maintenance over time.

[3] See footnote 2.

5.4   FDA- and AIFA-Approved Drugs for Chronic Weight Management

5.4.1   Orlistat

After the withdrawal from the US market of sibutramine, at present orlistat is the only drug available for chronic management of obesity in the United States and Europe. This was also the decision of the Italian Medicines Agency (AIFA). In Italy, as in several other countries, orlistat, in the formulation of 60 mg three times a day (TID), is available as over-the-counter drug (OTC). Some European countries have recently requested to reconsider the benefit/risk assessment for this drug [5]. The European Medicines Agency and the European drug regulatory (EMA) reconfirmed the positive benefit/risk ratio for orlistat.

Orlistat is a pancreatic lipase inhibitor that is taken as a tablet with meals and results in reduced fat absorption by the digestive tract, leading to increased fecal fat excretion. The reduction of ingested fat absorption is dose dependent. At a maximal dosage of 120 mg three times per day, up to 30 % of ingested fat is excreted [6].

A number of clinical trials have demonstrated increased weight loss and reduced weight regain with orlistat as compared with placebo. The mean weight loss difference between orlistat and placebo at 12 months is 2.89 kg [7]. Orlistat lowers hemoglobin A_{1c} and serum lipids beyond what can be explained by weight loss alone [8, 9].

Orlistat is generally well tolerated, and the occurrence of side effects in the gastrointestinal tract, such as cramps, flatulence with borborygmi, fatty stools, and fecal incontinence, is mainly due to inadequate adherence to dietary suggestions. Orlistat also reduces fat-soluble vitamin absorption due to its effects on fat absorption. Thus, supplementation of vitamins A, D, and E may be prudent. Given its excellent safety profile, orlistat is recommended for drug therapy of obese patients with cardiovascular disease, diabetes, and dyslipidemia.

5.5   FDA-Approved, EMA-Not-Approved Drugs for Management of Obesity

The US Food and Drug Administration has recently approved new prescription weight loss drugs: lorcaserin, and two-drug combination phentermine-topiramate. *Lorcaserin* activates the serotonin 2C receptor in the brain, helping a patient eat less and feel full after eating small amounts of food. The safety and efficacy of lorcaserin were evaluated in three randomized, placebo-controlled trials that included nearly 8000 obese and overweight patients, with and without type 2 diabetes, treated for 52–104 weeks [10–12]. Because in 1997, the weight loss drugs fenfluramine and dexfenfluramine were withdrawn from the market after evidence of heart valve damage due to activation of the serotonin 2B receptor on heart tissue, specific studies were conducted with the new drug. When used at the approved dosage of 10 mg twice a day, lorcaserin does not activate the serotonin 2B receptor. The most common side effects in nondiabetic patients are headache, dizziness, fatigue, nausea, dry mouth, and constipation and in diabetic patients are hypoglycemia, headache, back pain, cough, and fatigue.

Phentermine and topiramate is a combination of two FDA-approved drugs, phentermine and topiramate, in an extended-release formulation. Phentermine is indicated for short-term weight loss in overweight or obese adults; topiramate is indicated to treat certain types of seizures in people who have epilepsy and to prevent migraine headaches. The safety and efficacy of this drug combination were evaluated in two randomized, placebo-controlled trials that included approximately 3700 obese and overweight patients with and without significant weight-related conditions treated for 1 year [13–15]. The recommended daily dose contains 7.5 mg of phentermine and 46 mg of topiramate extended release. Regular monitoring of heart rate is recommended for all patients, especially when starting or increasing the dose.

5.6 FDA- and EMA-Approved Drugs for Management of Obesity

Liraglutide 3 mg and naltrexone – bupropion – were approved for patients with a BMI 30 kg/m^2 or more or for patients with a BMI of 27 kg/m^2 or more and comorbidity.

Liraglutide is a glucagon-like peptide-1 (GLP-1) receptor agonist with 97 % amino acid sequence homology to endogenous human GLP-1(7–37). GLP-1 is a physiological regulator of appetite and calorie intake, and the GLP-1 receptor is present in several areas of the brain involved in appetite regulation. Liraglutide lowers body weight through decreased calorie intake; its effect on the 24-h energy expenditure must be confirmed in obese patients. Liraglutide should not be used in combination with any other drug belonging to this class. Liraglutide 3 mg (brand name Saxenda) was approved by FDA for obesity treatment in December 2014. The safety and effectiveness of Saxenda were evaluated in three clinical trials that included approximately 4800 obese and overweight patients with and without significant weight-related conditions [16]. Dosing of liraglutide: inject subcutaneously (any time of day); initiate at 0.6 mg per day for the 1st week. At weekly intervals, increase the dose by 0.6 mg until a dose of 3.0 mg is reached. Response evaluation: stop if <4 % weight loss at 16 weeks. The percentage of patients with obesity or overweight with comorbidity achieving >5 % loss of body weight with liraglutide at 1 year is 62.3 % vs. 34.4 % for placebo. The percentage of patients achieving >10 % loss of body weight with liraglutide at 1 year is 33.9 % vs. 15.4 % for placebo.

The most frequent drug-related side effects are mild to moderate: transient nausea, constipation, fatigue, vomiting, and diarrhea; these side effects are clearly dose related, and it is likely that differences in subjects sensitivity to GLP-1 may be responsible for these effects. Serious side effects rarely reported in patients treated with this drug include pancreatitis and gallbladder disease. Liraglutide should be used cautiously in renal impairment, and it is also needed to monitor depression or suicidal thoughts. It can also slightly raise heart rate and should be discontinued in patients who experience a sustained increase in resting heart rate. Furthermore, liraglutide is contraindicated in patients with personal or family history of medullary thyroid carcinoma or multiple endocrine neoplasia syndrome type 2 [17].

Overall, liraglutide, with diet and exercise, produced sustained weight loss over 2 years in all studies and was not associated with major safety issues.

A combination of *naltrexone and bupropion* extended release was licensed by FDA in 2014 (brand name Contrave) and also received marketing authorization from the European Medicines Agency in March 2015 (under its European trade name, Mysimba). Bupropion is an antidepressant that enhances both noradrenergic and dopaminergic neurotransmission via reuptake inhibition. It is indicated for the treatment of depression, prevention of seasonal depressive disorder, and smoking cessation. Naltrexone is a pure opioid antagonist indicated for the treatment of alcohol dependence and for prevention of relapse to opioid dependence [18]. Bupropion stimulates hypothalamic pro-opiomelanocortin (POMC) neurons that release α-melanocyte-stimulating hormone (α-MSH) and β-endorphin; α-MSH binds to melanocortin 4 (MC4) receptors inhibiting food intake as well as increasing energy expenditure. On the contrary, binding of β-endorphin to μ-opioid receptors on POMC neurons mediates an autoinhibitory feedback loop leading to a decrease in the release of α-MSH. Naltrexone can antagonize the effects of β-endorphins and thereby interrupting the negative feedback loop. The coadministration of the two compounds thus leads to a more potent and prolonged stimulation of POMC neurons leading to synergistic effects on energy balance [19]. Naltrexone-bupropion combination was tested in four phase III trials involving more than 4500 overweight and obese people [20]. Dosing of bupropion-naltrexone: orally, 1 tab (8/90 mg) in am for 1 week, 1 in am and 1 in pm for 1 week, 2 in am and 1 in pm for 1 week, and 2 in am and 2 in pm. Response evaluation: stop if <5 % loss at 12 weeks.

The percentage of patients with obesity or overweight with comorbidity achieving >5 % loss of body weight with naltrexone-bupropion extended release (32/360 mg) at 1 year is 48 % vs. 16 % for placebo. The percentage of patients achieving >10 % loss of body weight at 1 year is 25 % vs. 7 % for placebo [20].

Side effects included nausea, headaches, constipation, dizziness, vomiting, diarrhea, and a dry mouth. Due to the presence of bupropion in the combination, the extended release formulation carries a black box warning indicating increased risk of suicidal behavior and ideation [21, 22]. The EMA said that uncertainty remained with regard to cardiovascular outcomes in the longer term, in spite of the extra study, whose interim results were "reassuring" [23].

References

1. EMA/808179/2009, EMA/H/A-10//1256 del 21/01/2010
2. EMEA/39457/2009 del 30/01/2009
3. Kaya A et al (2004) Efficacy of sibutramine, orlistat and combination therapy on short-term weight management in obese patients. Biomed Pharmacother 58:582–587

4. Douketis JD et al (2007) Systematic review of long-term weight loss studies in obese adults: clinical significance and applicability to clinical practice. Int J Obes (Lond) 31:1554–1559
5. European Medicines Agency. European Medicines Agency starts review of orlistat-containing medicines. http://www.ema.europa.eu/docs/en_GB/document_library/Press_release/2011/09/WC500112798.pdf
6. Zhi J et al (1994) Retrospective population-based analysis of the dose-response (fecal fat excretion) relationship of orlistat in normal and obese volunteers. Clin Pharmacol Ther 56:82–85
7. Li Z et al (2005) Meta-analysis: pharmacologic treatment of obesity. Ann Intern Med 142: 532–546
8. Hollander PA et al (1998) Role of orlistat in the treatment of obese patients with type 2 diabetes. A 1-year randomized double-blind study. Diabetes Care 21:1288–1294
9. Davidson MH et al (1999) Weight control and risk factor reduction in obese subjects treated for 2 years with orlistat: a randomized controlled trial. JAMA 281:235–242
10. Fidler MC, Sanchez M, Raether B et al (2011) A one-year randomized trial of lorcaserin for weight loss in obese and overweight adults: the BLOSSOM trial. J Clin Endocrinol Metab 96:3067–3077
11. Smith SR, Weissman NJ, Anderson CM et al (2010) Multicenter, placebo-controlled trial of lorcaserin for weight management. N Engl J Med 363:245–256
12. O'Neil PM, Smith SR, Weissman NJ et al (2012) Randomized placebo controlled clinical trial of lorcaserin for weight loss in type 2 diabetes mellitus: the BLOOM-DM study. Obesity 20:1426–1436
13. Garvey WT, Ryan DH, Look M et al (2012) Two-year sustained weight loss and metabolic benefits with controlled-release phentermine/topiramate in obese and overweight adults (SEQUEL): a randomized, placebo-controlled, phase 3 extension study. Am J Clin Nutr 95:297–308
14. Gadde KM, Allison DB, Ryan DH et al (2011) Effects of low-dose, controlled-release, phentermine plus topiramate combination on weight and associated comorbidities in overweight and obese adults (CONQUER): a randomised, placebo-controlled, phase 3 trial. Lancet 377: 1341–1352
15. Allison DB, Gadde KM, Garvey WT et al (2012) Controlled-release phentermine/topiramate in severely obese adults: a randomized controlled trial (EQUIP). Obesity (Silver Spring) 20:330–342
16. Astrup A, Carraro R, Finer N et al (2012) Safety, tolerability and sustained weight loss over 2 years with the once-daily human GLP-1 analog, liraglutide. Int J Obes (Lond) 36:843–854
17. Saxenda Vs. Liraglutide 3.0 mg label. http://www.accessdata.fda.gov/drugsatfda_docs/label/2014/206321Orig1s000lbl.pdf. Accessed 7 July 2015
18. Brunton L, Chabner BA, Knollman B (2011) Goodman and Gilman's the pharmacological basis of therapeutics, 12th edn. McGraw Hill Education, New York, 1808 p
19. Ornellas T, Chavez B (2011) Naltrexone SR/bupropion SR (Contrave). Pharmacol Ther 36(5):255–262
20. Greenway FL, Fujioka K, Plodkonski RA, et al; COR I Study Group (2010) Effect of naltrexone plus bupropion on weight loss in overweight and obese adults (COR-I): a multicentre, randomised, double-blind, placebo-controlled, phase 3 trial. Lancet 376:595–605
21. Takeda Pharmaceuticals America, Inc. Contrave (naltrexone HCl and bupropion Hcl) Extended-release tablets [package insert revised 9/2014] (2014) Orexigen Therapeutics, La Jolla
22. Mysimba summary of product characteristics (2015) http://www.ema.europa.eu/docs/en_GB/document_library/EPAR_-_Product_Information/human/003687/WC500185580.pdf. Accessed 26 May 2015
23. Hawkes N (2014) Approval of antiobesity drug is "major regression for patients' safety", says health watchdog. BMJ 349:g7805

Bariatric Surgery

6

Luca Busetto, Luigi Angrisani, Maurizio De Luca, Pietro Forestieri, Paolo Millo, and Ferruccio Santini

Bariatric surgery should be considered in the management of adult patients (age range 18–60 years) with severe obesity (BMI >40 kg/m^2 or BMI >35 kg/m^2 with comorbid conditions) who failed to lose weight or to maintain long-term weight loss, despite appropriate nonsurgical medical care, and are willing to participate in a postoperative long-term follow-up program. (*Level of evidence II, Strength of recommendation A*)

Bariatric surgery is contraindicated in patients with one of the following conditions: absence of a period of identifiable medical management, inability to participate in a prolonged medical follow-up, major psychiatric disorders if

L. Busetto (✉)
Department of Medicine, University of Padova, Padova, Italy
e-mail: luca.busetto@unipd.it

L. Angrisani
Laparoscopic, Emergency and General surgery, "S. Giovanni Bosco" Hospital, Napoli, Italy

M. De Luca
General Surgery, Montebelluna Hospital, Montebelluna (TV), Italy

P. Forestieri
Department of General Surgery, University "Federico II", Napoli, Italy

P. Millo
General Surgery, Aosta Regional Hospital, Aosta, Italy

F. Santini
Endocrinology Unit, University of Pisa, Pisa, Italy

© Springer International Publishing Switzerland 2016
P. Sbraccia et al. (eds.), *Clinical Management of Overweight and Obesity: Recommendations of the Italian Society of Obesity (SIO)*,
DOI 10.1007/978-3-319-24532-4_6

not otherwise indicated by their caring psychiatrist, alcohol and/or drug abuse, reduced life expectancy, and inability to care for themselves without adequate family or social support. (*Level of evidence VI, Strength of recommendation A*)

Bariatric surgery can be considered in the management of adolescents with BMI >35 kg/m^2 and serious comorbidities (type 2 diabetes mellitus, moderate or severe obstructive sleep apnea, pseudotumor cerebri, and severe steato-hepatitis) or with BMI>40 kg/m^2 and another comorbidity. Moreover, all the following inclusion criteria need to be satisfied: Tanner stage IV or V; skeletal maturation almost completed; ability to understand what dietary and physical activity changes will be required for optimal postoperative outcome; evidence of mature decision making, with appropriate understanding of potential risks and benefits of surgery; evidence of appropriate social support without evidence of abuse or neglect; appropriate treatment of possible coexisting psychiatric conditions; evidence that family and patient have the ability and motivation to comply with recommended treatments pre- and postoperatively. (*Level of evidence II, Strength of recommendation B*)

Bariatric surgery can be considered in the management of patients with severe obesity and age >60 years only after a careful individual estimate of risks and benefits, of potential improvement of the quality of life, and of the risk of mortality in the short-medium period. The primary aim of surgery in the elderly should be an improvement in quality of life and functional independence. (*Level of evidence IV, Strength of recommendation B*)

Available data are at present insufficient to support the general application of bariatric surgery in patients with a BMI lower than the cutoff reported by current guidelines. Nevertheless, there is no current justification to refuse access to bariatric surgery on simple BMI value in patients with mild obesity (BMI 30–35 kg/m^2) and severe comorbidities, in particular type 2 diabetes mellitus, who do not achieve a substantial weight reduction with nonsurgical methods. (*Level of evidence II, Strength of recommendation A*)

Bariatric surgery should be performed in clinical centers having the needed requirements: multidisciplinary team formed by dedicated medical and nonmedical personnel with specific knowledge and training, capability of performing diagnostic work-up and selection of the patients according to established guidelines, predefined surgical volume, technical facilities adequate to the assistance of patients with morbid obesity, postoperatory follow-up, management of early and late complications. (*Level of evidence VI, Strength of recommendation A*)

Preoperatory evaluation should include a routine preoperatory evaluation, as used for any major abdominal surgery, and the following specific evaluations: endocrinologic, diabetologic, cardiovascular, respiratory, gastroenterologic, and psychologic/psychatric. The assessment of nutritional status is important for the prevention of postoperative nutritional complications. (*Level of evidence V and VI, Strength of recommendation A*)

Reduction of the risk of surgery can be maximized with an optimal preoperatory control of comorbidities, the induction of a preoperative weight loss, and the use of adequate thrombo-embolic and antibiotic prophylaxis. (*Level of evidence I and VI, Strength of recommendation A*)

Surgical operations currently supported by good level of evidence studies with high number of patients and high rate of follow-up are as follows:

- Adjustable gastric banding
- Vertical banded gastroplasty
- Sleeve gastrectomy
- Gastric bypass
- Gastric bypass with single anastomosis or mini gastric bypass
- Biliopancreatic diversion
- Biliopancreatic diversion with duodenal switch. (*Level of evidence V, Strength of recommendation B*)

The laparoscopic approach is the first choice in bariatric surgery. The laparoscopic approach is advantageous compared to open surgery in terms of improving postoperative course and reducing complications. (*Level of evidence I, Strength of recommendation A*)

There is currently no evidence to indicate a particular bariatric procedure for any individual patient. The factors that have been proposed to be useful for the choice of the operation are factors related to the patient (age; sex; severity of obesity; fat distribution; body composition; complications and comorbidities, with particular reference to type 2 diabetes mellitus; life expectancy; quality of life; socioeconomic and cultural status; motivation; family and environmental support; geographical distance from the place of care), factors related to surgical technique (difficult technical implementation, results, short-term and long-term specific complications), and factors related to the surgeon (technical difficulties, culture and generic and specific experience, level of the hospital) (*Level of evidence VI, Strength of recommendation B*).

An organized and long-lasting follow-up should be offered to all bariatric patients, ideally for all their life. Follow-up should include diagnosis and management of all the adverse events related to surgery and management of comorbidities and complications (*Level of evidence VI, Strength of recommendation A*).

6.1 Clinical Management of Overweight and Obesity, Recommendations of the Italian Society of Obesity Bariatric surgery – Comments

6.1.1 Indications and Contraindications for Bariatric Surgery

6.1.1.1 Bariatric Surgery in Adults

In a 1991 NIH consensus conference on bariatric surgery, an expert panel released a statement on the criteria for patient selection [1]. Those guidelines have been repeatedly and even recently confirmed in international (ACC/AHA/TOS 2013; NICE 2014; IFSO-EC/EASO 2014) [2–4] and national frameworks (SICOB 2006) [5]. The criteria included in the 1991 guidelines are the following:

1. BMI >40 kg/m^2 (or BMI >35 kg/m^2 with comorbid conditions)
2. Age from 18 to 60 years
3. Obesity lasting >5 years
4. Failure to lose weight or to maintain long-term weight loss, despite appropriate nonsurgical medical care
5. Willingness to participate in a postoperative multidisciplinary treatment program

Comorbid conditions for which patients with BMI 35–40 kg/m^2 can be considered for bariatric surgery are those that significantly contribute to morbidity and mortality in obese patients, and in which surgically induced weight loss is expected to improve the disorder (such as metabolic disease, cardiorespiratory disease, severe joint disease, etc.). A recognized failure of previous nonsurgical treatment program may not be strictly required in patients with extremely high BMI (>50 kg/m^2) [3]. As for BMI criterion, it is important to note that a documented previous high BMI should be considered, meaning that weight loss as a result of intensified preoperative treatment is not a contraindication for the planned bariatric surgery, even if patients reach a BMI below that required for surgery. Furthermore, bariatric surgery is indicated in patients who exhibited a substantial weight loss following a conservative treatment program but started to regain weight [4].

The strength of '91 indications was confirmed by the results obtained in long-term controlled studies, the main one being the Swedish Obese Subjects (SOS) study, a controlled study that compared the outcome of 2000 patients who underwent bariatric surgery by various techniques with that of a matched control group that received conventional treatment [6]. In the surgery group, after 10 years, the average weight loss from baseline stabilized at 16.1 %, whereas in control subjects the average weight during the observation period increased by 1.6 %. This substantial difference in weight loss was associated with a higher remission rate of metabolic disease; a highly significant reduction of the incidence of new cases of diabetes; a reduction of cardiovascular events, both fatal and nonfatal; and a reduction of the incidence of new cases of cancer in women. Finally, during a follow-up to 10 years, the cumulative overall mortality in the surgery group was significantly lower than that observed in control subjects (RR: 0.76; 95 % CI: 0.59–0.99) [7]. The reduction in overall mortality in severely obese patients treated by bariatric surgery as compared with comparable subjects not surgically treated was confirmed by some retrospective studies [8–12], and by a recent meta-analysis (RR = 0.55; 95 % CI: 0.49–0.63) [13]. In conclusion, these results provide sufficient evidence that modern bariatric surgery can bring down the increased mortality observed in severely obese patients, provided that the perioperative mortality is maintained at low levels as reported in various studies (<0.5 %). The superiority of bariatric surgery over lifestyle intervention for weight loss and metabolic improvement has been confirmed by some randomized, controlled, clinical trials specifically performed in severely obese patients with type 2 diabetes mellitus. Dixon et al. randomized obese patients (BMI 30–40 kg/m^2) with recently diagnosed type 2 diabetes mellitus to gastric banding or conventional therapy with a focus on weight loss. At 2-year follow-up, remission of diabetes was achieved in 73 % patients in the surgical group and 13 % in the conventional therapy group [14]. Schauer et al. randomized obese patients (BMI 27–43 kg/m^2) with uncontrolled type 2 diabetes to receive either intensive medical therapy alone or intensive medical therapy plus Roux-en-Y gastric bypass or sleeve gastrectomy. The primary end-point was a glycated hemoglobin level of 6.0 % or less. At 3 years, the target was achieved in 5 % of the patients in the medical therapy group, as compared with 38 % of those in the gastric bypass group and 24 % of those in the sleeve gastrectomy group. Both weight loss and glycemic control were greater in the surgical groups than in the medical therapy group [15]. Mingrone et al. randomly assigned obese patients (BMI >35 kg/m^2), with a history of at least 5 years of diabetes and a glycated hemoglobin level of ≥7.0 %, to receive conventional medical therapy or undergo either gastric bypass or biliopancreatic diversion. At 2 years, no diabetes remission occurred in the medical therapy group, while it was observed in 75 % patients from the gastric bypass group and 95 % from the biliopancreatic diversion group [16]. Finally, Ikramuddin et al. randomized obese diabetic patients (BMI 30–40 kg/m^2) to receive intensive medical management or Roux-en-Y gastric bypass plus intensive lifestyle-medical management protocol. The primary end-point was a composite goal of HbA1c less than 7.0 %, low-density lipoprotein cholesterol less than 100 mg/dL, and systolic blood pressure less than 130 mmHg. At 12 months, this goal was achieved in 49 % patients in the gastric bypass group and in 19 % patients in the lifestyle-medical management group [17]. A direct comparison among these four studies is made difficult by differences in inclusion criteria, primary procedures, and definition of therapeutic goals, but the overall message is a confirmation of the superiority of bariatric surgery over medical therapy in producing an improvement of metabolic control and/ or achieving remission of type 2 diabetes in the obese patient.

Contraindications for bariatric surgery reported in the '91 document, and constantly confirmed thereafter, can be summarized as follows:

1. Absence of a period of identifiable medical management
2. Patients who are unable to participate in prolonged medical follow-up
3. Psychotic disorders, severe depression, personality and eating disorders, as evaluated by a psychiatrist or a psychologist with specific expertise in obesity (unless specifically advised by these team experts)
4. Alcohol abuse and/or drug dependencies
5. Diseases threatening life in the short term
6. Patients who are unable to care for themselves and have no adequate family or social support

In the presence of severe psychopathologic diseases, bariatric surgery is in general terms contraindicated, unless suggested by exceptional circumstances related to severe medical conditions (fatal prognosis related to the obese state), and always with the approval of the reference psychiatrist [18].

6.1.1.2 Bariatric Surgery in Adolescents

The NIH '91 guidelines did not suggest the use of bariatric surgery in severely obese subjects of age <18 years [1], and the surgical practice in young patients has been limited for a long time. The Interdisciplinary European Guidelines, in agreement with the recommendations of a consensus document of American pediatricians [19], suggest more stringent criteria than those applied to the adults:

1. BMI >40 kg/m^2 (or 99.5th percentile for respective age) and at least one comorbidity

2. A follow-up period of at least 6 months of adequate medical therapy of obesity in a specialized center
3. Skeletal and developmental maturity
4. Ability to commit to comprehensive medical and psychological evaluation before and after surgery
5. Motivation to participate in a postoperative multidisciplinary treatment program
6. Ease of access to a unit with specialist pediatric support

However, under the pressure of the boost of obesity in young people, the application of bariatric surgery to adolescents is progressively increasing, and its results have been submitted to a careful and complete review [20]. The results of a randomized, controlled, clinical trial that compared bariatric surgery (gastric banding) with a lifestyle intervention program in a small group of adolescents of 14–18 years and BMI >35 kg/m^2 confirmed the superiority of bariatric surgery at 2-year follow-up in terms of weight loss and improvement of comorbidities and quality of life [21]. On the base of this novel knowledge, it is nowadays reasonable to move the indications for bariatric surgery in adolescents near to those used in adults. The selection criteria that have been recently proposed are the following [20]:

1. BMI >35 kg/m^2 and serious comorbidities (type 2 diabetes mellitus, moderate or severe obstructive sleep apnea (AHI >15 events/h), pseudotumor cerebri, and severe steatohepatitis)
2. BMI >40 kg/m^2 and another comorbidity (mild obstructive sleep apnea (AHI ≥5 events/h), hypertension, insulin resistance, glucose intolerance, dyslipidemia, impaired quality of life, or activities of daily living)
3. Tanner stage IV or V (unless severe comorbidities indicate bariatric surgery earlier)
4. Skeletal maturity completed at least 95 % of estimated growth
5. Ability to understand what dietary and physical activity changes will be required for optimal postoperative outcomes
6. Evidence of mature decision making, with appropriate understanding of the potential risks and benefits of surgery
7. Evidence of appropriate social support without evidence of abuse or neglect
8. Appropriate treatment of possible coexisting psychiatric conditions (depression, anxiety, or binge eating disorder).
9. Evidence that family and patient have the ability and motivation to comply with recommended treatments pre- and postoperatively, including consistent use of micronutrient supplements; evidence may include a history of reliable attendance at office visits for weight management and compliance with other medical needs

The procedures that have collected enough evidence to be recommended in adolescents are gastric bypass [20] and gastric banding [21]. It is recommended that bariatric surgery in adolescents is performed in highly specialized centers with extensive multidisciplinary experience and pediatric surgical skills [4].

6.1.1.3 Bariatric Surgery in Patients Aged Over 60 Years

The NIH '91 guidelines did not suggest the use of bariatric surgery in severely obese subjects of age>60 years [1]. However, there are in literature reports of elderly subjects treated by bariatric surgery, which show satisfactory results [22–27]. Generally, these studies regard patients between 60 and 70 years in a good clinical and physical function and report a greater incidence of postoperative complications and a lower weight loss as compared to those that regard younger patients, yet displaying advantages in terms of improvement or remission of comorbid conditions as well as amelioration of functional autonomy and quality of life. Ultimately, bariatric surgery can be taken into consideration in patients of age >60 years, with indications similar to those applied in the adult patients, after careful individual estimate of risks and benefits, of potential improvement of the quality of life, and of the risk of mortality in the short-medium period [28].

6.1.1.4 Bariatric Surgery in Patients with BMI 30–35 kg/m^2

The superiority of bariatric surgery over a lifestyle-medical management program in inducing weight loss and improving comorbid conditions has been demonstrated also in patients with moderate obesity (BMI 30–35 kg/m^2) by a small randomized, controlled trial with a 2-year follow-up [29]. Furthermore, patients with BMI <35 kg/m^2 were included in 3 of the 4 clinical randomized, controlled trials performed in obese patients with type 2 diabetes, which have shown that surgical therapy was more effective than conventional therapy in terms of metabolic control and remission of diabetes [14, 15, 17]. The recognition of a major effect of bariatric surgery on metabolic control in type 2 diabetic patients finally suggested the use of conventional surgical procedures in diabetic patients with lower BMI (BMI 30–35 kg/m^2 or even BMI 25–30 kg/m^2) and the introduction of new procedures, such as ileal interposition and duodenal-jejunal exclusion, designed with the specific goal of obtaining a favorable metabolic effect without inducing a major weight loss. The results of bariatric surgery, either performed by conventional procedures or experimental techniques, in diabetic patients with BMI <35 kg/m^2 have been recently appraised by some meta-analyses and systematic reviews [30, 31]. Li et al. have recently completed a large meta-analysis of both prospective and retrospective, nonrandomized studies concerning the metabolic effects of surgery in diabetic patients with BMI <35 kg/m^2, including a total of 13 studies and 357 treated patients [30]. Reis et al. performed a review of the literature on the role of bariatric and metabolic surgery in diabetic patients with BMI <35 kg/m^2, including 29 studies and 1209 patients [31]. Overall, the results of these studies indicated a satisfactory remission of diabetes at short-medium term in patients with BMI 30–35 kg/m^2, whereas it was not as good in patients with BMI 25–30 kg/m^2. This trend has been confirmed by Scopinaro et al. [32] in a prospective study of biliopancreatic diversion. At present, however, there are no results in the long term describing the risk/benefit ratio of bariatric surgery in patients with moderate obesity (with or without diabetes), and the potential risks related to excessive weight loss should be considered with caution in this category of patients.

Recently, the 2014 ADA Standards of Medical Care in Diabetes [33] confirmed that although small trials have shown glycemic benefit of bariatric surgery in patients with type 2 diabetes and BMI 30–35 kg/m², there is currently insufficient evidence to generally recommend surgery in patients with BMI <35 kg/m². A broader position has been taken by the IDF that suggests to consider bariatric surgery in type 2 diabetic patients with BMI 30–35 kg/m² when diabetes cannot be adequately controlled by optimal medical regimen, especially in the presence of other major cardiovascular disease risk factors [34]. According to the 2013 clinical practice guidelines of the American Association of Clinical Endocrinologists, the Obesity Society, and the American Society for Metabolic and Bariatric Surgery, patients with BMI of 30–34.9 kg/m² with diabetes or metabolic syndrome may also be offered a bariatric procedure, although current evidence is limited by the number of subjects studied and lack of long-term data demonstrating net benefit [35]. The Clinical Issue Committee of the American Society for Metabolic and Bariatric Surgery highlighted the results of recent randomized clinical trials, already described, and recommended that for patients with BMI 30–35 kg/m² who do not achieve substantial and durable weight and comorbidity improvement with nonsurgical methods, bariatric surgery should be an available option [36]. Application of bariatric surgery to diabetic patients with BMI 30–35 kg/m² has also been suggested for people with recent onset type 2 diabetes (NICE 2014) [3] or on an individual basis (IFSO-EC/EASO 2014) [4]. Finally, a recent position statement from the International Federation for the Surgery of Obesity and Metabolic Disorders regarding bariatric surgery in class I obesity highlighted the inadequacy of the simple BMI value as an indicator of the clinical state and of the comorbidity burden in the obese patient; it emphasized that patients with relatively low BMI values may have a comorbidity burden similar to, or greater than, patients with more severe obesity and concluded that denial of bariatric surgery to obese patients with BMI 30–35 kg/m² suffering from severe comorbidities and not achieving weight control with nonsurgical therapy does not appear to be clinically justified [37].

In conclusion, available data are insufficient to support the safety profile and efficacy of bariatric surgery in patients with a BMI lower than the cutoff reported by current guidelines. Nevertheless, there is no current justification to refuse access to bariatric surgery on simple BMI value to patients with mild obesity (BMI 30–35 kg/m²) and severe comorbidities, in particular type 2 diabetes mellitus, who do not achieve a substantial weight reduction with nonsurgical methods.

6.1.2 Preoperatory Evaluation and Preparation for Surgery

6.1.2.1 Requirements for a Bariatric Surgery Center

Bariatric surgery is one of the possible therapeutic options in obesity management. Bariatric surgery should be therefore performed in clinical centers having the possibility to offer to the patients an adequate diagnostic work-up for obesity and related comorbidities and the possibility to engage also nonsurgical treatments for obesity. Bariatric surgery should be performed in dedicated surgical units having the needed surgical expertise and skills. Minimal requirements for building a bariatric surgery center are the following [3]:

1. Multidisciplinary team formed by dedicated medical and nonmedical personnel with specific knowledge and training
2. Diagnostic work-up and selection of the patients according to established guidelines
3. Predefined surgical volume
4. Technical facilities adequate to the assistance of patients with morbid obesity
5. Postoperatory follow-up
6. Management of early and late complications

The multidisciplinary team (physician expert in obesity management, psychologist or psychiatrist, dietician, bariatric surgeon, and anesthesiologist) represents according to all guidelines [1–5] a fundamental requirement of the center, allowing a complete approach to the obese patient. The team should collaborate in patient selection, choice of the surgical technique, management of complex cases requiring specific interventions, follow-up. Logistically, the center needs to have the technical facilities necessary for a safe and proper assistance to the patient with morbid obesity. These include the facilities in the outpatient offices, in the ward, in the operatory room and the diagnostic facilities. The center needs to have direct access to a postoperatory intensive care unit.

6.1.2.2 Preoperatory Evaluation

Preoperatory evaluation should be performed by a dedicated multidisciplinary team (physician expert in obesity management, psychologist or psychiatrist, dietician, bariatric surgeon, and anesthesiologist). All candidates for bariatric surgery should undergo a routine preoperatory evaluation, as used for any major abdominal surgery, and the following specific tests [35, 38–44]:

1. *Endocrinologic evaluation* for the exclusion of endocrine disorders causing obesity or requiring a specific management and correction before surgery. Determination of thyroid and adrenocortical functions should be performed in all cases, and further endocrine evaluations (pituitary, parathyroid, gonadal function) should be done in case of specific disturbances.
2. *Diabetologic evaluation*, even in the absence of diabetes history, with determination of fasting blood glucose and glycated hemoglobin and execution of an oral glucose tolerance test with glucose and insulin measurements.
3. *Cardiovascular evaluation* with standard EKG in all cases and further diagnostic tests (echocardiography, Holter EKG, stress tests) in case of clinical data suggesting the presence of a cardiac disease.
4. *Respiratory evaluation* with spirometry and arterial blood gas analysis in patients with known respiratory problems. The execution of a polysomnography or a cardiorespiratory sleep study is mandatory in case of diurnal or nocturnal symptoms suggestive of sleep respiratory disturbances. Patients having moderate-to-severe sleep apnea syndrome should be adapted to nocturnal ventilation before surgery.
5. *Gynecologic-mammographic screening* for endometrial and breast cancer.
6. *Abdominal ultrasound.* Obesity is associated with a higher prevalence of gallbladder disease, and the rapid weight loss following surgery further predis-

poses to gallstone formation. Italian guidelines for bariatric surgery suggest the execution of an abdominal ultrasound for gallstone detection in all patients with consensual colecistectomy in patients found to have gallstones [5]. Nonalcoholic fatty liver disease (NAFLD) is another important obesity-related comorbidity. Abdominal ultrasound detects the presence and the severity of NAFLD and can show evolution of NALD to liver fibrosis and cirrhosis. The evolution to cirrhosis should be carefully considered, both for the risk of esophageal bleeding and for the possible negative effects of a rapid weight loss on liver function.

7. *Esophago-gastro-duodenoscopy (EGDS)*. The need for a routine endoscopic study of the first gastrointestinal tract before bariatric surgery is still debated [43]. However, several considerations are in favor of routine preoperatory EGDS. The presence of a gastroesophageal reflux disease, a large hiatal ernia, gastric lesions, Barrett esophagus, Helicobacter infection could require specific treatment or could influence the choice of the surgical procedure [5]. Considering these considerations and according to other clinical practice guidelines [45], the recommendation for a routine endoscopic study before surgery appears to be reasonable.

8. *Psycologic/psychiatric evaluation*. Morbid obesity is associated with a higher prevalence of psycopathology (depression, anxiety, eating behavior disturbances, personality disorders), and about half of the patients who are candidates for bariatric surgery use psychoactive drugs [46]. The evaluation of the mental status of the obese patients is necessary for the indication to undergo bariatric surgery, and it is important for the choice of the surgical procedure [18, 43, 47, 48].

9. *Nutritional evaluation*. The knowledge of the eating behaviors and habits of the obese candidate for bariatric surgery is important for the choice of the type of bariatric procedures [43, 46]. The evaluation of the preoperatory nutritional status is important for the prevention of postoperatory nutritional complications. A preoperative weight loss program is recommended in order to reduce surgical risks.

6.1.2.3 Preparation for Surgery

Comorbidities Control
An optimal control of the comorbidities before surgery is highly recommended, with a particular reference to those comorbidities known to influence the surgical risk (optimization of the pharmacologic treatment in patients with type 2 diabetes and hypertension; adaptation to the nocturnal ventilation in patients with moderate-to-severe sleep apnea syndrome) [35, 42].

Preoperatory Weight Loss
A preoperatory weight loss equal to about 10–15 % of the initial body weight is able to produce a substantial reduction in liver volume in nonrandomized studies [49–52]. This level of weight loss has been also associated with important improvements in respiratory function and respiratory sleep disturbances in patients with severe visceral obesity [53]. These relevant anatomic modifications can facilitate the surgical and anesthesiological management of the patients during surgery and reduce the risk of complications, as indicated in a nonrandomized controlled retrospective study comparing patients with severe visceral obesity having or not having had a

preoperatory weight loss [54]. Both very low calorie diet (VLCD) [49–51] and the application of an intragastric balloon have been used for the induction of the preoperatory weight loss in bariatric patients [52–54].

Prevention of Thrombo-Embolic Complications
Obese candidates for bariatric surgery should be considered at high risk for thrombo-embolic disease and should therefore receive mechanical and pharmacologic preventive measures. Several prophylactic regimes are available, but some specific points remain controversial (choice of the anticoagulant, dose and duration of the treatment, etc.). Pharmacologic prophylaxis should be started immediately after surgery and continued for at least 2–4 weeks. Clinical experience demonstrates that the use of mechanical and pharmacologic preventive measures greatly reduces, but not completely prevents, thrombo-embolic complications [43, 55–57].

Antibiotic Prophylaxis
Several studies identified obesity as a risk factor for surgical wound infections. Antibiotic prophylaxis should be done in bariatric surgery using the same scheme applied in major abdominal surgery, with adjusting of the dose according to the weight of the patient [58, 59].

6.1.3   Surgical Techniques and Criteria for the Choice of the Operation

6.1.3.1 Surgical Techniques
Surgical operations currently supported by good level of evidence studies with high number of patients and high rate of follow-up are as follows:

- Adjustable gastric banding
- Vertical banded gastroplasty
- Sleeve gastrectomy
- Gastric bypass
- Gastric bypass with single anastomosis or mini gastric bypass
- Scopinaro biliopancreatic diversion
- Biliopancreatic diversion with duodenal switch

Gastric Banding
Gastric banding consists in the placement of a band with a pneumatic internal chamber around the upper part of the stomach. The band is applied under the gastro-esophageal junction and creates a small pouch (25 ml). The chamber is connected to a silicone connecting tube ending with a reservoir placed subcutaneously on the abdominal wall and allows a percutaneous adjustment of the size of the band. Gastric banding does not change permanently the anatomy of the stomach, and it is therefore completely reversible. Gastric banding has the purpose of slowing down the meal, inducing a feeling of rapid satiety after the introduction of small quantities of food. The patient may be gradually accustomed to the presence of the banding by

exploiting the possibility of calibration of the shrinkage. The operative complications are very rare (0.2 %), and the operative mortality is very low (<0.1 %). The main postoperative complications are represented by migration of the band within the stomach (<1 %), gastric pouch dilatation and stomach slippage (3 %), disconnection of the port and/or connecting tube with leakage of the system (3 %). Results in terms of weight loss are around 40–50 % of excess weight. Long-term results are related to the eating behavior of the patient, and there is a significant number of patients with some degree of weight regain [60–65].

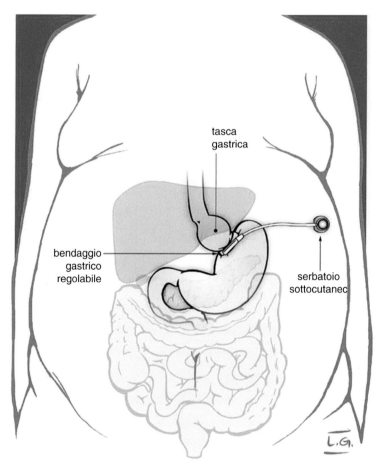

Vertical Banded Gastroplasty

It is one of the oldest restrictive operations. It consists in the partition and reduction of the stomach in order to create a small proximal gastric pouch (15–20 ml) in communication with the gastric remnant through a small passage restricted by a polypropylene mesh. The mechanism of action is similar to the band, but there is not the possibility to calibrate the mesh. Operative mortality is low (0.1 %). Main postoperative specific complications are represented by stenosis of the outlet (1–2 %), gastric pouch dilatation, and gastroesophageal reflux (1 %). The results in terms of weight loss are evaluated around 60–70 % of excess weight. Even in case of vertical gastroplasty, long-term results are dependent on the eating behavior of the patient and there is a significant number of cases with weight regain. For this reason and for the fact that similar results can be obtained with less invasive restrictive procedures, vertical banded gastroplasty is now almost abandoned [66].

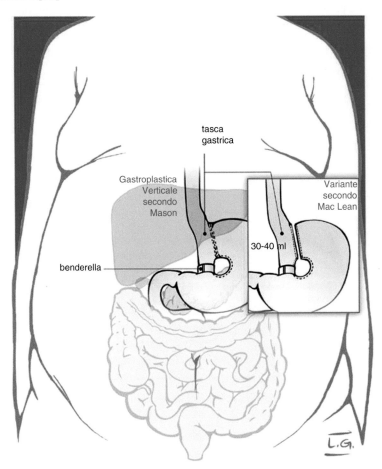

Sleeve Gastrectomy

This is a partially restrictive procedure consisting in the section of the stomach with removal of approximately 2/3 of it. The section takes place parallel to the small curvature in order to create a stomach in a tubular form. The operation reduces drastically the amount of food that can be ingested and causes a feeling of early satiety. However, the removal of a significant part of the stomach and/or modification of the speed of gastric transit also causes changes in the secretion of hormones secreted in the gastrointestinal tract and having a regulatory action on energy balance and carbohydrate metabolism. Sleeve gastrectomy was initially introduced as a first step of a more complex operation (duodenal switch) in patients with severe cardiorespiratory problems and with high BMI, but is now also proposed as a single operation. Operative mortality is about 0.2 %, and it is frequently related to leaks at the level of the long gastric suture. Main postoperative specific complications are represented by dilatation of the pouch and gastroesophageal reflux. The results in terms of weight loss can be evaluated at around 60–70 % of excess weight. Long-term results are good, but there is a significant number of cases in which patients show at least partial weight regain. In these cases, the second step (duodenal switch) or another redo procedure might be indicated [67–71].

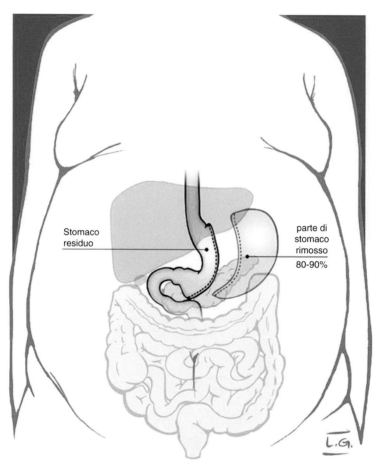

Stomaco residuo

parte di stomaco rimosso 80-90%

L.G.

Gastric Bypass

This operation consists in the creation of a proximal gastric pouch (15–20 cc) which is excluded from the gastric remnant. The small pouch is sutured to the jejunum through a Roux-en-Y intestinal derivation. The stomach and the duodenum are excluded from the transit of the food. Weight loss occurs in part through a restrictive mechanism and also as the result of the modification of the secretion of entero-acting hormones regulating energy balance and glucose metabolism. The presence of a dumping syndrome following the intake of beverages and/or sweet foods can also participate in the determination of the weight loss. There is not a significant malabsorption of macronutrients (fat, carbohydrates, proteins), but there is a certain degree of malabsorption for some micronutrients (Ca, Fe, and vit B12). The operative complications are about 2 %, and the operative mortality is about 0.5 %. The main postoperative specific complications are represented by anastomotic leak (1 %), anastomotic stenosis (1.5 %), anastomotic ulcer (3 %), internal hernias (3 %). Possible nutritional complications are represented by multifactorial anemia (more frequently microcytic iron deficiency anemia) and osteoporosis/osteomalacia. The prevention of complications requires nutritional supplements of vitamins and minerals that should be adapted to the needs of the patients. The results in terms of weight loss are evaluated around 55–65 % of excess weight. Weight loss is rapid in the first year. The changes in the secretion of the enteroinsular hormones allow a rapid and specific effect of improvement of metabolic control in patients with type 2 diabetes mellitus [60, 72–75].

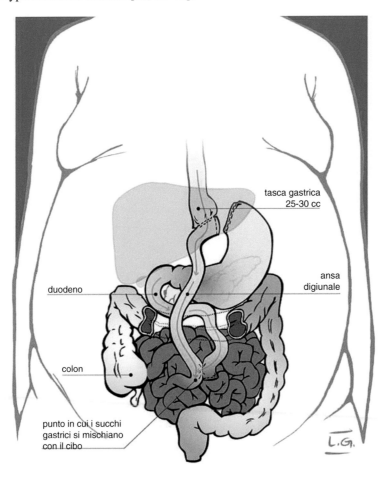

Single Anastomosis Gastric Bypass or Mini Gastric Bypass

Single anastomosis gastric bypass or mini gastric bypass was introduced in 1997 in order to simplify and possibly reduce the risk of classic gastric bypass, creating a reversible procedure with possibility of conversion to another surgery. Some authors define this procedure Billroth II gastric bypass or Omega loop gastric bypass or BAGUA. The operation consists in a long, narrow gastric tubulization along the lesser curvature of the stomach that is anastomosed to a very long jejunal loop. The mini gastric bypass can be considered a technique with a restrictive action caused by gastric tubulization and a moderate malabsorption caused by the exclusion of 180–250 cm of small intestine from the transit of the food. The gastric tubulization along the lesser curvature is long enough to be compared by some authors to a sleeve gastrectomy. The benefits appear to consist in a greater technical simplicity and lower rate of perioperative complications compared to gastric bypass, with good results in terms of long-term weight loss and remission of diabetes and comorbidities. Perioperative complications are around 1.7 %. In particular, they are the gastrojejunal anastomosis fistula (0.9 %), fistula of the gastric suture of the pouch (0.2 %), fistula of the gastric remnant (0.2), stenosis of the gastrojejunal anastomosis (0.2 %), bleeding of the suture line or gastrojejunal anastomosis (0.2 %). Long-term complications are perianastomotic ulcer (0.6 %) and reflux esophagitis (1.5 %). Studies show weight loss at 5 years of 75 % of excess weight and good maintenance even at 10 years. Remission of diabetes is approximately 85 % of cases. Prevention of nutritional complications requires continuous supplementation with multivitamins, calcium, vitamin D, vitamin B12, and iron even after the mini gastric bypass [76–82].

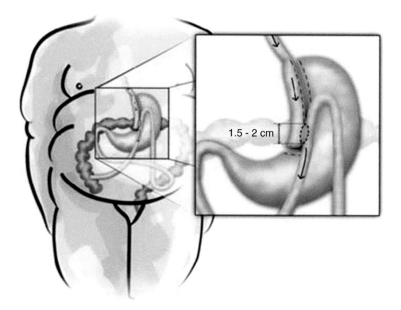

Biliopancreatic Diversion

This operation, invented by Nicola Scopinaro, is a predominantly malabsorptive proce-dure and consists in the reduction of the volume of the stomach by subtotal gastrec-tomy and in the preparation of a gastrojejunal anastomosis creating an alimentary loop of 200 cm, a 50-cm common channel from the ileocecal valve, and a long biliopancre-atic loop. Scopinaro biliopancreatic diversion causes malabsorption of some nutrients, especially dietary fat. Surgical complications are about 5 %, and operative mortality is about 1 %. Main specific surgical postoperative complications are represented by post-anastomotic peptic ulcer (3.4 %), anastomotic stenosis, occlusion of the biliary/diges-tive loop, internal hernias. Nutritional complications, related to the mechanism of action of the operation, are more frequent than in the gastric bypass and include pro-tein-energy malnutrition, multifactorial anemia, bone demineralization, deficits of fat-soluble vitamins. The prevention of nutritional complications requires an adequate nutritional intake of proteins and a continuous or periodic long-lasting supplementation of multivitamins, calcium, vitamin D, vitamin B12, and iron. Frequent symptoms are related to the malabsorption (diarrhea, halitosis, smelly flatulence) and proctologic complications (hemorrhoids, anal abscesses and fistulas). Results in terms of weight loss are evaluable around 65–75 % of the excess weight and are very stable in time. Enteroinsular hormone changes, together with fat malabsorption, allow a very impres-sive improvement of metabolic control in patients with type 2 diabetes [60, 83–88].

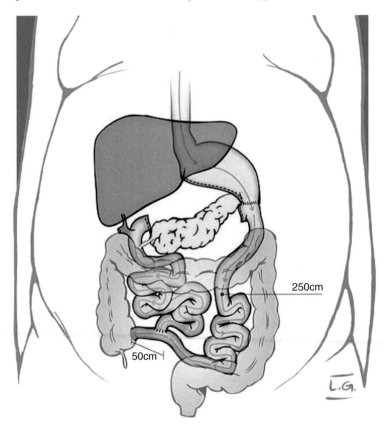

Biliopancreatic Diversion Duodenal Switch

This is a variant of the classic biliopancreatic diversion consisting in the partial reduction of the volume of the stomach (with a sleeve gastrectomy), in the preservation of the pylorus and the first 3–4 cm of the duodenum, and in the preparation of a gastroduodenal anastomosis creating an alimenatry loop of 200 cm, a 50-cm common channel from the ileocecal valve, and a long biliopancreatic loop. Mechanism of action, mortality, late complications, and nutritional and surgical results are similar to those obtained with the classical biliopancreatic diversion [60, 89–91].

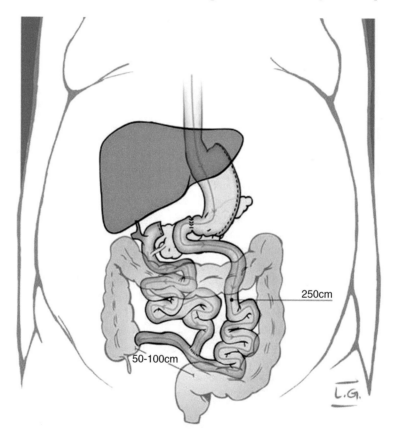

In Italy, other surgical operations are also currently used that cannot be considered sufficiently standardized (biliary-intestinal bypass, Amenta-Cariani functional gastric bypass, Vassallo SuperMagen-strasse, Furbetta functional gastric bypass, duodenal-ileal bypass anastomosis with single sleeve gastrectomy, gastric plication) for their limited use to a few centers and/or for the inadequate follow-up (time or number of patients) [92–97]. Some investigational endoscopic bariatric treatments are in the phase of development and investigation (intragastric adjustable implantable prosthesis, endoscopic gastroplasty, duodenal-jejunal sleeve [98, 99], procedures involving gastric electrical stimulation, or vagal blockade [100–102]). New procedures are designed with the aim to induce the metabolic effects of surgery without causing a significant weight loss (duodenal-jejunal bypass, ileal transposition) [103–105]. Among the future perspectives, new possibilities can be offered to bariatric surgery by NOTES (natural orifice transluminal endoscopic surgery), SILS (single-incision laparoscopic surgery) [106], and the use of robotics [107].

Laparoscopy in Bariatric Surgery
All the bariatric surgical procedures have been done by laparoscopy. The laparoscopic approach is the first choice in bariatric surgery. Data from prospective randomized studies have shown that the laparoscopic approach is advantageous compared to open surgery in terms of improved postoperative course and reduced complications [108–112].

6.1.3.2 Criteria of Choice of the Bariatric Operation
The various types of operation, as well as having different mode of action, provide different results in terms of weight loss and have specific advantages and specific complications, presenting a risk/benefit ratio in many ways different. Randomized trials comparing procedures [113] largely confirm these differences, but do not solve the problem, substantially again highlighting the mutual benefits and disadvantages. An assessment of the risk/benefit ratio in general terms is therefore extremely difficult and largely subjective. In agreement with other European and national guidelines, it can be said that there is currently no evidence to indicate a particular bariatric procedure for any individual patient [4–5]. The factors that have been proposed to be useful for the choice of operation in the individual patient are factors related to the patient (age; sex; severity of obesity; fat distribution; body composition; complications and comorbidities, with particular reference to type 2 diabetes mellitus; life expectancy; quality of life; socioeconomic and cultural status; motivation; family and environmental support; geographical distance from the place of care), factors related to surgical technique (difficult technical implementation, results, short-term and long-term specific complications), and factors related to the surgeon (technical difficulties, culture and generic and specific experience, level of the hospital). However, there is no uniformity of views regarding the role of these factors in determining the technical choice.

6.1.4   The Role of the Intragastric Balloon

The intragastric balloon is a silicone prosthesis that can be inserted in the stomach for a limited lapse of time (usually 6 months) and that can therefore cause a temporary artificial feeling of gastric filling facilitating the caloric restrictions. The placement and the following removal take place in endoscopy and usually in deep sedation. Controlled randomized studies have shown that the intragastric balloon allows in the 6 months of its application a weight loss superior than that achievable through a low-calorie diet [114]. The balloon is usually well tolerated even though side effects can appear: dyspepsia and persistent vomiting with the necessity of premature removal (1 %), gastric erosions (0.2 %), esophagitis (1.3 %), and spontaneous breakage with the risk of distal migration and intestinal occlusion (0.4 %) [115]. Reports show isolated incidents of mortality for gastric perforation in patients with previous gastric surgery [115]. The main problem, linked to the transience of the device, is represented by the following weight regain, even though a part of the weight loss can be maintained in a significant percentage of patients [116]. A more rational indication for the intragastric balloon is its use as a mean for achieving a substantial preoperative weight loss in those super obese patients who are suitable candidates for bariatric surgery or for other surgery but who present a very high obesity-related anesthesiological risk [54].

6.1.5   Follow-Up

6.1.5.1   General Follow-Up for Bariatric Surgery
An organized and long-lasting follow-up should be offered to all bariatric patients. Follow-up should include diagnosis and management of all the adverse events related to surgery and management of comorbidities and complications. Multidisciplinary outpatient control visits, both surgical and nonsurgical, should be scheduled for all patients possibly reducing the number of accesses to the center [4, 5]. Time schedule generally recommended comprehends clinical and laboratory controls every 3 months in the first year after surgery and every 6–12 months thereafter [5]. This follow-up schedule should be offered to all patients, including patients with good clinical status and weight loss.

Nutritional Prescriptions
Patients should remain fasting in the early postoperative period (24–72 h depending on the type of procedure), eventually with a nasogastric tube inserted, until the normal canalization of the upper gastrointestinal tract has been checked with a radiologic examination. A short course of liquid diet (form first to third postoperative days) is prescribed after all bariatric procedure, followed by a period (2–4 weeks) of a semiliquid morbid diet. Patients should receive detailed instructions on the modalities of reintroduction of solid food at the moment of discharge or at the first month postoperative visit [35, 42, 43]. Nutritional prescriptions should be continuously reinforced during follow-up, in particular after pure restrictive procedures, and also in all the procedures involving a reduction of the gastric volume (sleeve gastrectomy, gastric bypass) [35, 42, 43]. Patients should be educated to maintain a protein intake of at least 1.5 g/kg of ideal body weight (eventually as protein supplements) and, immediately after the postoperative period, to engage in at least 30 minutes per day of mixed (aerobic and resistance) physical activity, in order to reduce the loss of fat-free mass [35, 42, 43].

Drug Treatments
The use of proton pump inhibitors is advisable in the first period after all bariatric procedures. The pharmacologic management of comorbidities (type 2 diabetes, hypertension) should be periodically reevaluated. Patients should receive detailed instructions about vitamin supplementation [35, 39, 40, 117].

Endoscopic and/or Radiologic Control

A postoperatory endoscopic and/or radiologic control should be done after any type of bariatric procedure. Further endoscopic and/or radiologic controls should be guided by the occurrence of specific symptoms or in case of suspected complications [35, 39, 40, 117].

Failures

Several studies showed that a proportion of patients treated with bariatric surgery did not achieve a good weight loss or regain weight. In case of partial failure, the introduction in the bariatric management of behavioral therapy or drugs can be helpful. In case of failure, a redo surgery should be considered.

Redo Surgery

The global rate of redo surgery after bariatric procedures reported in the literature ranges between 5 % and 50 %. Indications for the conversion of a bariatric procedure are the following: (1) poor weight loss, (2) anatomic complications (gastric pouch dilatation, sleeve dilatation, etc.), (3) eating behaviors not adequate to the mechanism of action of the bariatric procedure or changes of eating behavior during the follow-up. Among bariatric procedures, the operation with the lower rate of redo surgery is biliopancreatic diversion (5 %), with increasing rate of revision in gastric bypass (10–20 %); vertical banded gastroplasty (25–55 %); and gastric banding (40–50 %). The existence of a group of nonresponders to bariatric surgery should be also considered: patients showing poor weight loss or weight regain despite maximal efforts by the surgeon and the multidisciplinary team. Several studies demonstrated that weight loss after redo surgery is in general lower than observed after primary bariatric procedures. Randomized trials suggesting validated algorithms for clinical decision in redo surgery are not available, and therefore the clinical decision is largely based on the surgeon's experience and the global evaluation by the multidisciplinary team. Redo bariatric surgery has a rate of intraoperative major complications definitely higher than primary bariatric surgery. Therefore, redo surgery should be performed in highly specialized bariatric centers [5, 118–121].

Plastic Surgery

The important weight loss observed after bariatric surgery can cause the formation of skin excess and localized residual adipose tissue depots, in particular at the level of the abdomen and upper and lower limbs. These aesthetic problems can also interfere with activities of daily living and cause psychological distress to the patients. A plastic surgeon with expertise in postbariatric body weight remodeling should be a part of the multidisciplinary team. The proper timing for plastic surgery should be decided by the multidisciplinary team. Reconstructive plastic surgery should be considered as an integral part of the bariatric treatment, and it should be therefore covered by public health system.

6.1.5.2 Follow-Up Notes Specific for the Single Bariatric Procedure

Adjustable Gastric Banding

Postoperatory adjustments of the banding should be performed according to weight loss, eating behavior, and gastric side effects and decided by the multidisciplinary team. Adjustments of the banding should be done under radiologic guidance, with the exclusion of the first adjustments for bandings with large volumes and low inflation pressures [122]. In gastric banding, a pure restrictive procedure, continuous long-term routine vitamin supplementation is not mandatory.

Vertical Banded Gastroplasty and Sleeve Gastrectomy

Nutritional recommendations are similar to those used for gastric banding, with the obvious exception of the postoperatory adjustment that is not feasible. Cases of "Dumping Syndrome" (see above) have been described after sleeve gastrectomy. The continuous use of an oral vitamin supplementation is warranted, and the possibility of long-term vitamin B12 deficit should be considered [35, 39, 40].

Gastric Bypass

A routine oral supplementation of vitamins and micronutrients (calcium included) should be prescribed for all the life of the patients. Supplementation with high and/ or parenteral doses of specific micronutrients (calcium and iron) can be needed in case of documented deficits. Laboratory follow-up should include the evaluation of the nutritional status (hemoglobin, iron, ferritin, vitamin B12, folate, vitamin D, PTH, calcium, magnesium). "Dumping Syndrome" can occur when the gastrointestinal remodeling causes a rapid gastric emptying and the rapid passage of the undigested alimentary bolus in the small bowel. Dumping is characterized by the abrupt onset of vagal symptoms and by the later tendency to hypoglycemia, caused by the activation of the enteroinsular endocrine axis (incretins). Patients should be made aware of the symptoms of the syndrome, should be able to recognize it, and should be informed about the nutritional-behavioral changes that can help the prevention of dumping (adequate hydration before meals and use of fiber supplements). Pharmacologic treatment or redo surgery may be rarely needed in case of severe symptoms. In case of lactose intolerance, the use of lactase supplements can be useful. The use of proton pump inhibitors (PPI) is advisable in the first year after surgery [35, 39, 40].

Biliopancreatic Diversion

A routine oral supplementation of vitamins (including fat-soluble vitamins) and micronutrients (included calcium at least 2 g/day) should be prescribed for all the life of the patients, in order to compensate for the malabsorption. Supplementation with high and/or parenteral doses of specific micronutrients (calcium and iron, fat-soluble vitamins) can be needed in case of documented deficits. Laboratory follow-up should include the evaluation of the nutritional status (hemoglobin, iron, ferritin, vitamin B12, folate, vitamin D, PTH, calcium, magnesium, zinc, copper). A high-protein intake (at least 90 g/day) is strongly advisable in order to prevent protein-calories malnutrition. The use of PPI is advisable in the first year after surgery. Gastroenteric side effects (bloating, flatulence, smelly feces, diarrhea) can be controlled with neomycine or metronidazole and/or pancreatic enzymes [35, 39, 40].

References

1. Gastrointestinal surgery for severe obesity (1991) National Institutes of Health Consensus Development Conference draft Statement. Obes Surg 1:257–266
2. American College of Cardiology/American Heart Association Task Force on Practice Guidelines/Obesity Expert Panel (2014) Executive Summary: guidelines (2013) for the management of overweight and obesity in adults. A report of the American College of Cardiology/American Heart Association Task Force on Practice Guidelines and The Obesity Society.
3. National Institute for Health and Clinical Excellence. Obesity: identification, assessment and management of overweight and obesity in children, young people and adults. NICE clinical guideline 189. Nov 2014
4. Fried M, Yumuk V, Oppert JM et al (2014) on behalf of International Federation for the Surgery of Obesity and Metabolic Disorders – European Chapter (IFSO-EC) and European Association for the Study of Obesity (EASO). Interdisciplinary European Guidelines on Metabolic and Bariatric Surgery. Obes Surg 24:42–55
5. Società Italiana di Chirurgia dell'Obesità e delle malattie metaboliche (2006) Linee guida e stato dell'arte della chirurgia bariatrica e metabolica in Italia. SICOB 1–87
6. Sjöström L (2013) Review of the key results from the Swedish Obese Subjects (SOS) trial – a prospective controlled intervention study of bariatric surgery. J Intern Med 273:219–234
7. Sjöström L, Narbro K, Sjöström CD et al (2007) Swedish Obese Subjects Study: Effects of bariatric surgery on mortality in Swedish obese subjects. N Engl J Med 357:741–752
8. MacDonald KG Jr, Long SD, Swanson MS et al (1997) The gastric bypass operation reduces the progression and mortality of non-insulin-dependent diabetes mellitus. J Gastrointest Surg 1:213–220
9. Christou NV, Sampalis JS, Liberman M et al (2004) Surgery decreases long-term mortality, morbidity, and health care use in morbidly obese patients. Ann Surg 240:416–423
10. Adams TD, Gress RE, Smith SC et al (2007) Long-term mortality after gastric bypass surgery. N Engl J Med 357:753–761
11. Busetto L, Mirabelli D, Petroni ML et al (2007) Comparative long-term mortality after laparoscopic adjustable gastric banding versus nonsurgical controls. Surg Obes Relat Dis 3: 496–502
12. Peeters A, O'Brien PE, Laurie C et al (2007) Substantial intentional weight loss and mortality in the severely obese. Ann Surg 246:1028–1033
13. Pontiroli AE, Morabito A (2011) Long-term prevention of mortality in morbid obesity through bariatric surgery. A systematic review and meta-analysis of trials performed with gastric banding and gastric bypass. Ann Surg 253:1–4
14. Dixon JB, O'Brien PE, Playfair J et al (2008) Adjustable gastric banding and conventional therapy for type 2 diabetes: a randomized controlled trial. JAMA 299:316–323
15. Schauer PR, Bhatt DL, Kirwan JP et al (2014) Bariatric surgery versus intensive medical therapy for diabetes – 3-Year outcomes. N Engl J Med 370:2002–2013
16. Mingrone G, Panunzi S, De Gaetano A et al (2012) Bariatric surgery versus conventional medical therapy for type 2 diabetes. N Engl J Med 366:1577–1585
17. Ikramuddin S, Korner J, Lee WJ et al (2013) Roux-en-Y Gastric Bypass vs intensive medical management for the control of type 2 diabetes, hypertension, and hyperlipidemia. The Diabetes Surgery Study randomized clinical trial. JAMA 309:2240–2249

18. Busetto L, Cerbone MR, Lippi C, Micanti F, Sampietro S. Società Italiana di Chirurgia dell'Obesità e delle Malattie Metaboliche (2011) Suggerimenti per la valutazione psicologico-psichiatrica del paziente obeso candidato alla chirurgia bariatrica. SICOb
19. Inge TH, Krebs NF, Garcia VF et al (2004) Bariatric surgery for severely overweight adolescents: concerns and recommendations. Pediatrics 114:217–223
20. Pratt JSA, Lenders CM, Dionne EA et al (2009) Best practice updates for pediatric/adolescent weight loss surgery. Obesity 17:901–910
21. O'Brien PE, Sawyer SM, Laurie C et al (2010) Laparoscopic adjustable gastric banding in severely obese adolescents. A randomized trial. JAMA 303:519–526
22. Sugerman HJ, DeMaria EJ, Kellum JM et al (2004) Effects of bariatric surgery in older patients. Ann Surg 240:243–247
23. Quebbemann B, Engstrom D, Siegfried T et al (2005) Bariatric surgery in patients older than 65 years is safe and effective. Surg Obes Relat Dis 1:389–392
24. Hazzan D, Chin EH, Steinhagen E et al (2006) Laparoscopic bariatric surgery can be safe for treatment of morbid obesity in patients older than 60 years. Surg Obes Relat Dis 2:613–616
25. Taylor CJ, Layani L (2006) Laparoscopic adjustable gastric banding in patients > or = 60 years old: is it worthwhile? Obes Surg 16:1579–1583
26. Dunkle-Blatter SE, St Jean MR, Whitehead C et al (2007) Outcomes among elderly bariatric patients at a high-volume center. Surg Obes Relat Dis 3:163–169
27. Busetto L, Angrisani L, Basso N et al (2008) Safety and efficacy of laparoscopic adjustable gastric banding in the elderly. Obesity 16:334–338
28. Villareal DT, Apovian CM, Kushner RF, Klein S (2005) Obesity in older adults: technical review and position statement of the American Society for Nutrition and NAASO, The Obesity Society. Am J Clin Nutr 82:923–934
29. O'Brien PE, Dixon JB, Laurie C et al (2006) Treatment of mild to moderate obesity with laparoscopic adjustable gastric banding or an intensive medical program. A randomized trial. Ann Intern Med 144:625–633
30. Li Q, Chen L, Yang Z et al (2012) Metabolic effects of bariatric surgery in type 2 diabetic patients with bodymass index of 35 kg/m2. Diabetes Obes Metab 14:262–270
31. Reis CEG, Alvarez-Leite JI, Bressan J et al (2012) Role of bariatric–metabolic surgery in the treatment of obese type 2 diabetes with body mass index <35 kg/m2: a literature review. Diabetes Technol Ther 14:365–372
32. Scopinaro N, Adami GF, Papadia FS et al (2011) The effects of biliopancreatic diversion on type 2 diabetes mellitus in patients with mild obesity (BMI 30–35 kg/m^2) and simple overweight (BMI 25–30 kg/m^2): A prospective controlled study. Obes Surg 21:880–888
33. American Diabetes Association (2014) Standards of medical care in diabetes – 2014. Diabetes Care 37:S14–S80
34. Dixon JB, Zimmet P, Alberti KG et al (2011) Bariatric surgery: an IDF statement for obese type 2 diabetes. Diabet Med 28:628–642
35. Mechanick JI, Youdim A, Jones DB et al (2013) Clinical practice guidelines for the perioperative nutritional, metabolic, and nonsurgical support of the bariatric surgery patient—2013 update: cosponsored by American Association of Clinical Endocrinologists, the Obesity Society, and American Society for Metabolic and Bariatric Surgery. Surg Obes Relat Dis 9:159–191
36. Clinical Issues Committee ASMBS (2013) Bariatric surgery in class I obesity (BMI 30–35 kg/m2). Surg Obes Relat Dis 9:e1–e10
37. Busetto L, Dixon J, De Luca M, Shikora S, Pories W, Angrisani L (2014) Bariatric surgery in class I obesity. A position statement from the International Federation for the Surgery of Obesity and metabolic disorders (IFSO). Obes Surg 24:487–519
38. Ferraro DR (2004) Preparing patients for bariatric surgery-the clinical considerations. Clin Rev 14:57–63
39. Kelly J, Tarnoff M, Shikora S et al (2005) Best practice recommendations for surgical care in weight loss surgery. Obes Res 13:227–233
40. Saltzman E, Anderson W, Apovian CM et al (2005) Criteria for patient selection and multi-disciplinary evaluation and treatment of the weight loss surgery patient. Obes Res 13: 234–243

41. Heber D, Greenway FL, Kaplan LM et al (2010) Endocrine and nutritional management of the post-bariatric surgery patient: an Endocrine Society Clinical Practice Guideline. J Clin Endocrinol Metab 95:4823–4843
42. Mechanick JI, Kushner RF, Sugerman HJ et al (2009) American Association of Clinical Endocrinologists, The Obesity Society, and American Society for Metabolic & Bariatric Surgery medical guidelines for clinical practice for the perioperative nutritional, metabolic, and nonsurgical support of the bariatric surgery patient. Obesity 17:S1–S70
43. Tariq N, Chand B (2011) Presurgical evaluation and postoperative care for the bariatric patient. Gastrointest Endosc Clin N Am 21:229–240
44. Fierabracci P, Pinchera A, Martinelli S et al (2011) Prevalence of endocrine diseases in morbidly obese patients scheduled for bariatric surgery: beyond diabetes. Obes Surg 21:54–60
45. Sauerland S, Angrisani L, Belachew M et al (2005) European Association for Endoscopic Surgery: Obesity surgery: evidence-based guidelines of the European Association for Endoscopic Surgery (EAES). Surg Endosc 19:200–221
46. Dahl JK, Eriksen L, Vedul-Kjelsås E et al (2010) Prevalence of all relevant eating disorders in patients waiting for bariatric surgery: a comparison between patients with and without eating disorders. Eat Weight Disord 15:e247–e255
47. Piaggi P, Lippi C, Fierabracci P, Maffei M, Calderone A, Mauri M, Anselmino M, Cassano GB, Vitti P, Pinchera A, Landi A, Santini F (2010) Artificial neural networks in the outcome prediction of adjustable gastric banding in obese women. PLoS One 5:e13624
48. Pull CB (2010) Current psychological assessment practices in obesity surgery programs: what to assess and why. Curr Opin Psychiatry 23:30–36
49. Fris RJ (2004) Preoperative low energy diet diminishes liver size. Obes Surg 14:1165–1170
50. Edholm D, Kullberg J, Haenni A et al (2011) Preoperative 4-week low- calorie diet reduces liver volume and intrahepatic fat, and facilitates laparoscopic gastric bypass in morbidly obese. Obes Surg 21:345–350
51. Lewis MC, Phillips ML, Slavotinek JP et al (2006) Change in liver size and fat content after treatment with Optifast® Very Low Calorie Diet. Obes Surg 16:697–701
52. Frutos MD, Morales MD, Luján J et al (2007) Intragastric balloon reduces liver volume in superobese patients, facilitating subsequent laparoscopic gastric bypass. Obes Surg 17:150–154
53. Busetto L, Enzi G, Inelmen EM et al (2005) Obstructive sleep apnea syndrome in morbid obesity: effects of intragastric balloon. Chest 128:618–623
54. Busetto L, Segato G, De Luca M et al (2004) Pre-operative weight loss by intragastric balloon in super obese patients treated with laparoscopic gastric banding: a Case-control study. Obes Surg 14:671–676
55. Geerts WH, Pineo GF, Heit JA et al (2004) Prevention of venous thromboembolism: the Seventh ACCP Conference on Antithrombotic and Thrombolytic Therapy. Chest 126:338S–400S
56. Gonzalez QH, Tishler DS, Plata-Munoz JJ et al (2004) Incidence of clinically evident deep venous thrombosis after laparoscopic Roux en-Y gastric bypass. Surg Endosc 18:1082–1084
57. Forestieri P, Quarto G, De Caterina M et al (2007) Prophylaxis of thromboembolism in bariatric surgery with parnaparin. Obes Surg 17:1558–1562
58. Wurtz R, Itokazu G, Rodvold K (1997) Antimicrobial dosing in obese patients. Clin Infect Dis 25:112–118
59. Pai MP, Bearden DT (2007) Antimicrobial dosing considerations in obese adult patients. Pharmacotherapy 27:1081–1091
60. Parikh MS, Laker S, Weiner M, Hajiseyedjavadi O, Ren CJ (2006) Objective comparison of complications resulting from laparoscopic bariatric procedures. J Am Coll Surg 202:252–261
61. Chapman AE, Kiroff G, Game P et al (2004) Laparoscopic adjustable gastric banding in the treatment of obesity: a systematic literature review. Surgery 135:326–351
62. Chevallier JM, Zinzindohoue F, Douard R et al (2004) Complications after laparoscopic adjustable gastric banding for morbid obesity: experience with 1,000 patients over 7 years. Obes Surg 14:407–414
63. Ponce J, Paynter S, Fromm R (2005) Laparoscopic adjustable gastric banding: 1,014 consecutive cases. J Am Coll Surg 201:529–535

64. O'Brien PE, McPhail T, Chaston TB, Dixon JB (2006) Systematic review of medium-term weight loss after bariatric operations. Obes Surg 16:1032–1040
65. Favretti F, Ashton D, Busetto L, Segato G, De Luca M (2009) The gastric band: first-choice procedure for obesity surgery. World J Surg 33:2039–2048
66. Morino M, Toppino M, Bonnet G, Rosa R, Garrone C (2002) Laparoscopic vertical banded gastroplasty for morbid obesity. Assessment of efficacy. Surg Endosc 16:1566–1572
67. Regan JP, Inabnet WB, Gagner M, Pomp A (2003) Early experience with two-stage laparoscopic Roux-en-Y gastric bypass as an alternative in the super-super obese patient. Obes Surg 13:861–864
68. Silecchia G, Boru C, Pecchia A et al (2006) Effectiveness of laparoscopic sleeve gastrectomy (first stage of biliopancreatic diversion with duodenal switch) on co-morbidities in super-obese high-risk patients. Obes Surg 16:1138–1144
69. Himpens J, Dapri G, Cadiere GB (2006) A prospective randomized study between laparoscopic gastric banding and laparoscopic isolated sleeve gastrectomy: results after 1 and 3 years. Obes Surg 16:1450–1456
70. Braghetto I, Korn O, Valladares H et al (2007) Laparoscopic sleeve gastrectomy: surgical technique, indications and clinical results. Obes Surg 17:1442–1450
71. Himpens J, Dobbeleir J, Peeters G (2010) Long-term results of laparoscopic sleeve gastrectomy for obesity. Ann Surg 25:319–324
72. Wittgrove AC, Clark GW (2000) Laparoscopic gastric bypass, Roux en-Y, 500 patients: technique and results with 3–60 months follow-up. Obes Surg 10:233–239
73. Higa KD, Boone KB, Ho T, Davies OG (2000) Laparoscopic Roux-en-Y gastric-bypass for morbid obesity: technique and preliminary results of our first 400 patients. Arch Surg 135:1029–1033
74. Nguyen NT, Rivers R, Wolfe BM (2003) Factors associated with operative outcomes in laparoscopic gastric bypass. J Am Coll Surg 197:548–555
75. Schauer PR, Burguera B, Ikramuddin S et al (2003) Effect of laparoscopic Roux-en Y gastric bypass on type 2 diabetes mellitus. Ann Surg 238:467–485
76. Rutledge R (2001) The mini-gastric bypass: experience with the first 1272 cases. Obes Surg 11:276–280
77. Lee WJ, Ser KH, Lee YC (2012) Laparoscopic Roux-en-Y versus mini-gastric bypass for the treatment of morbid obesity: a 10-year experience. Obes Surg 22:1827–1834
78. Kim Z, Hur KY (2011) Laparoscopic Mini Gastric Bypass for type 2 diabetes: the preliminary report. World J Surg 35:631–636
79. Caballero M, Carbajo M (2004) One Anastomosis Gastric Bypass: a simple, safe and efficient surgical procedure for treating morbid obesity. Nutr Hosp 19:372–375
80. Noun R, Zeidan S, Riachi E (2007) Mini Gastric Bypass for revision of failed primary restrictive procedures: a valuable option. Obes Surg 17:684–688
81. Chevallier JM, Chakhtoura G, Zinzindohouè F (2009) Laparoscopic mini gastric bypass. J Chir 146:60–64
82. Musella M, Susa A, Greco F, De Luca M, Manno E, Di Stefano C (2014) The laparoscopic mini-gastric bypass: the italian experience: outcomes from 974 consecutive cases in a multi-center review. Surg Endosc 28:156–163
83. Scopinaro N, Gianetta E, Civalleri D, Bonalumi U, Bachi V (1979) Bilio-pancreatic bypass for obesity: II. Initial experience in man. Br J Surg 66:618–620
84. Scopinaro N, Gianetta E, Adami GF et al (1996) Biliopancreatic diversion for obesity at eighteen years. Surgery 119:261–268
85. Scopinaro N, Marinari GM, Camerini G (2002) Laparoscopic standard biliopancreatic diversion: technique and preliminary results. Obes Surg 12:362–365
86. Scopinaro N, Marinari GM, Camerini GB, Papadia FS, Adami GF (2005) Specific effects of biliopancreatic diversion on the major components of metabolic syndrome: a longterm follow-up study. Diabetes Care 28:2406–2411
87. Marinari GM, Papadia FS, Briatore L, Adami G, Scopinaro N (2006) Type 2 diabetes and weight loss following biliopancreatic diversion for obesity. Obes Surg 16:1440–1444

88. Scopinaro N, Papadia F, Marinari G, Camerini G, Adami G (2007) Long-term control of type 2 diabetes mellitus and the other major components of the metabolic syndrome after biliopancreatic diversion in patients with BMI <35 kg/m2. Obes Surg 17:185–192
89. Marceau P, Hould FS, Simard S et al (1998) Biliopancreatic diversion with duodenal switch. World J Surg 22:947–954
90. Hess DS, Hess DW (1998) Biliopancreatic diversion with a duodenal switch. Obes Surg 8:267–282
91. Gagner M (2004) Laparoscopic biliopancreatic diversion with duodenal switch. Laparoscopic Bariatric Surgery. Lippincott Williams & Wilkins, Philadelphia, pp 133–142
92. Doldi SB, Lattuada E, Zappa MA et al (1998) Biliointestinal bypass: another surgical option. Obes Surg 8:566–570
93. Cariani S, Amenta E (2007) Three-year results of Roux-en-Y gastric bypass-on-vertical banded gastroplasty: an effective and safe procedure which enables endoscopy and X-ray study of the stomach and biliary tract. Obes Surg 17:1312–1318
94. Furbetta F, Gambinotti G (2002) Functional gastric bypass with an adjustable gastric band. Obes Surg 12:876–880
95. Vassallo C, Berbiglia G, Pessina A et al (2007) The Super-Magenstrasse and Mill operation with pyloroplasty: preliminary results. Obes Surg 17:1080–1083
96. Sánchez-Pernaute A, Herrera MA, Pérez-Aguirre ME et al (2010) Single anastomosis duodeno-ileal bypass with sleeve gastrectomy (SADI-S). One to three-year follow-up. Obes Surg 20:1720–1726
97. Talebpour M, Amoli BS (2007) Laparoscopic total gastric vertical plication in morbid obesity. J Laparoendosc Adv Surg Tech A 17:793–798
98. de Jong K, Mathus-Vliegen EM, Veldhuyzen EA, Eshuis JH, Fockens P (2010) Short-term safety and efficacy of the Trans-oral Endoscopic Restrictive Implant System for the treatment of obesity. Gastrointest Endosc 72:497–504
99. Schouten R, Rijs CS, Bouvy ND et al (2010) A multicenter, randomized efficacy study of the EndoBarrier Gastrointestinal Liner for presurgical weight loss prior to bariatric surgery. Ann Surg 251:236–243
100. De Luca M, Segato G, Busetto L et al (2004) Progress in implantable gastric stimulation: summary of results of the European multi-center study. Obes Surg 14:S33–S39
101. Sanmiguel CP, Conklin JL, Cunneen SA et al (2009) Gastric electrical stimulation with the TANTALUS System in obese type 2 diabetes patients: effect on weight and glycemic control. J Diabetes Sci Technol 3:964–970
102. Ikramuddin S, Blackstone RP, Brancatisano A et al (2014) Effect of reversible intermittent intra-abdominal vagal nerve blockade on morbid obesity: the ReCharge randomized clinical trial. JAMA 312:915–922
103. Cohen RV, Schiavon CA, Pinheiro JS, Correa JL, Rubino F (2007) Duodenal-jejunal bypass for the treatment of type 2 diabetes in patients withBMI 22–34: a report of two cases. Surg Obes Relat Dis 3:195–197
104. Ramos AC, Galvao Neto MP, de Souza YM et al (2009) Laparoscopic duodenaljejunal exclusion in the treatment of type 2 diabetes mellitus in patients with BMI <30 kg/m2. Obes Surg 19:307–312
105. De Paula AL, Stival AR, Macedo A et al (2010) Prospective randomized controlled trial comparing 2 versions of laparoscopic ileal interposition associated with sleeve gastrectomy for patients with type 2 diabetes with BMI 21–34 kg/m(2). Surg Obes Relat Dis 6:296–304
106. Tacchino RM, Greco F, Matera D, Diflumeri G (2010) Single-incision laparoscopic gastric bypass for morbid obesity. Obes Surg 20:1154–1160
107. Parini U, Fabozzi M, Brachet Contul R et al (2006) Laparoscopic gastric bypass performed with the Da Vinci Intuitive Robotic System: preliminary experience. Surg Endosc 20:1851–1857
108. De Luca M, de Werra C, Formato A et al (2000) Laparotomic vs laparoscopic lap-band: 4-year results with early and intermediate complications. Obes Surg 10:266–268
109. Davila-Cervantes A, Borunda D, Dominguez-Cherit G et al (2002) Open versus laparoscopic vertical banded gastroplasty: a randomized controlled double blind trial. Obes Surg 12:812–818

110. Kim WW, Gagner M, Kini S et al (2003) Laparoscopic vs. open biliopancreatic diversion with duodenal switch: a comparative study. J Gastrointest Surg 7:552–557
111. Lujan JA, Frutos MD, Hernandez Q et al (2004) Laparoscopic versus open gastric bypass in the treatment of morbid obesity: a randomized prospective study. Ann Surg 239:433–437
112. Hutter MM, Randall S, Khuri SF et al (2006) Laparoscopic versus open gastric bypass for morbid obesity. A multicenter, prospective, risk-adjusted analysis from the national surgical quality improvement program. Ann Surg 243:657–666
113. Nguyen NT, Slone JA, Nguyen XM, Hartman JS, Hoyt DB (2009) A prospective randomized trial of laparoscopic gastric bypass versus laparoscopic adjustable gastric banding for the treatment of morbid obesity: outcomes, quality of life, and costs. Ann Surg 250:631–641
114. Genco A, Cipriano M, Bacci V et al (2006) Bioenterics Intragastric Balloon: a short term, double blind, randomized, controlled, crossover study on weight reduction in morbidly obese patients. Int J Obes 30:129–133
115. Genco A, Bruni T, Doldi SB et al (2005) BioEnterics Intragastric Balloon: The Italian experience with 2,515 patients. Obes Surg 15:1161–1164
116. Mathus-Vliegen EM, Tytgat GN (2005) Intragastric balloon for treatment-resistant obesity: safety, tolerance, and efficacy of 1-year balloon treatment followed by a 1-year balloon-free follow-up. Gastrointest Endosc 61:19–27
117. Ziegler O, Sirveaux MA, Brunaud L, Reibel N, Quilliot D (2009) Medical follow up after bariatric surgery: nutritional and drug issues. General recommendations for the prevention and treatment of nutritional deficiencies. Diabetes Metab 35:544–557
118. Buhmann H, Vines L, Schiesser M (2014) Operative strategies for patients with failed primary bariatric procedures. Dig Surg 31:60–66
119. Brethauer SA, Kothari S, Sudan R et al (2014) Systematic review on reoperative bariatric surgery: American Society for Metabolic and Bariatric Surgery Revision Task Force. Surg Obes Relat Dis 10:952–972
120. Lannoo M, Dillemans B (2014) Laparoscopy for primary and secondary bariatric procedures. Best Pract Res Clin Gastroenterol 28:159–173
121. Kellogg TA (2011) Revisional bariatric surgery. Surg Clin North Am 91:1353–1371
122. Busetto L, Segato G, De Marchi F, Foletto M, De Luca M, Favretti F, Enzi G (2003) Postoperative management of laparoscopic gastric banding. Obes Surg 13:121–127

Metabolic-Nutritional- Psychological Rehabilitation in Obesity

7

Lorenzo Maria Donini, Amelia Brunani, Paolo Capodaglio,
Maria Grazia Carbonelli, Massimo Cuzzolaro,
Sandro Gentili, Alessandro Giustini, and Giuseppe Rovera

7.1 Recommendations

The rationale and the procedures of *Rehabilitation Medicine* can be optimally applied to the natural history of obesity, which is characterised by the presence of comorbidities, chronicity and disability with an important impact on quality of life. *Level of Evidence (LoE): I; Strength of the Recommendation (SoR): A*

L.M. Donini (✉)
Sapienza University of Rome, Italian Society for the Study of Eating Disorders, Rome, Italy
e-mail: lorenzomaria.donini@uniroma1.it

A. Brunani • P. Capodaglio
San Giuseppe Hospital, Istituto Auxologico Italiano Piancavallo, Verbania, Italy

M.G. Carbonelli
S. Camillo – Forlanini Hospital, Rome, Italy

M. Cuzzolaro
Sapienza University of Rome, Italian Society for the Study of Eating Disorders, Rome, Italy

Chief Eating & Weight Disorders, Italian Society for the Study of Eating Disorders, Rome, Italy

S. Gentili
Tor Vergata University of Rome, Rome, Italy

A. Giustini
San Pancrazio Hospital – Arco (Trento) – Eur Soc Phys Rehab Medicine, Rome, Italy

G. Rovera
San Luca Hospital, Turin – Italian Association of Food Science and Nutrition Specialists, Ponce, Puerto Rico

© Springer International Publishing Switzerland 2016
P. Sbraccia et al. (eds.), *Clinical Management of Overweight and Obesity: Recommendations of the Italian Society of Obesity (SIO)*,
DOI 10.1007/978-3-319-24532-4_7

The metabolic-nutritional-psychological rehabilitation is part of the health-*care network* for obese patient, and it includes outpatient /semi-residential (*day hospital, day service, diagnostic and therapeutic-rehabilitative community centre*) or residential facilities (*residential intensive rehabilitation (cod. 56), psychiatric rehabilitation*, therapeutic-rehabilitative communities*). Level of Evidence: VI; SoR:A*

The metabolic-nutritional-psychological rehabilitation represents a suitable *approach to obesity* when the level of the over-nutrition is severe, during the phases of instability of somatic and psychological comorbidities, when disability level is severe and quality of life significantly reduced. *Level of Evidence: VI; SoR:A*

During the multidimensional evaluation of obese subjects, quality of life, disability level, muscular function (muscular strength, balance, functional exercise capacity) and osteoarticular problems (pain, articular limitations) have to be assessed. *Level of Evidence: III; SoR:A*

The therapeutic-rehabilitative pathway of an obese patient must include, in an integrated approach, nutritional, rehabilitative and psycho-educational interventions together with rehabilitative nursing. *Level of Evidence: IV; SoR:A*

The *intensity* of the rehabilitative intervention must be related to the severity of disability and of comorbidities, to the psychological status and to the quality of life of the patient. *Level of Evidence: VI; SoR:A*

The rehabilitative pathway can play an essential role during the preparation of the patients to bariatric or plastic-reconstructive *surgery* and during the follow-up phase, in order to reduce the preoperative risks and to improve the results especially in the long term. *Level of Evidence: III; SoR:A*

> The access to intensive residential or semi-residential rehabilitation may be appropriate even in the absence of an acute event, based on the disability indexes and the clinical appropriateness for the obesity-specific rehabilitative treatment as assessed by:
>
> - TSD-RD: Test SIO for obesity-related disability
> - CASCO-R: Comprehensive Appropriateness Scale for the Care of Obesity in Rehabilitation. *Level of Evidence: III; SoR:A*

7.2   Comments

7.2.1   Clinical-Functional and Psychological Obesity and Disability

Somatic and psychological comorbidities, disability and quality of life in the different phases of life are the principal determinants leading to the progression of the clinical and functional phenotype of obesity [1–3].

Following the bio-psychosocial model of the *International Classification of Functioning, Disability and Health* (ICF) and the *core set* for obese patients, the authors highlighted the changes in several specific functional areas [4] where therapeutic rehabilitative programs are mandatory.

Quality of life Questionnaires (i.e. SF36) show an important negative effect of obesity not only on physical limitations but also on psychological discomfort and social behaviour.

Beyond the well-known medical complications, obesity is most of the time associated with a reduced psycho-physical well-being, eating disorder (in particular *binge eating disorder* or BED and *night eating syndrome* or NES), low self-esteem and depression [5–13].

In the last years, an independent relation between obesity and disability in activities of daily living (ADL = OR 2.2 in men and 2.4 in women) due to increased body mass and obesity-related symptoms (pain, dyspnea, sleeping disorders) has been shown [14]. It has been also reported that, in addition to a reduction in life expectancy, obese people suffer from a substantial reduction of years without disability (5.7 for men and 5.02 for women) [15]. These evidences call for rehabilitative and social interventions beyond the available medical (diet therapy, drugs) and surgical treatments [15].

Literature suggests a hierarchy in the appearance of the obesity-related disability: the first functions affected are those related to the lower limbs (strength and balance) because in human bipedal stance they are keys for independence and appear more vulnerable when compared to the upper limb ones (strength and manual ability) [16].

Obesity is growing considerably among elderly people (>65 years): in this age group, the effects on disability related to obesity and ageing sum up together [17–22]. The combined effects due to obesity and the physiological depletion of lean mass (sarcopenia) are more relevant than the effects of the two factors separately [19].

Obese subjects experience "hostile" medical, cultural and occupational [23] situations. This stigma is associated with a higher risk of depression and with a reduction of self-esteem, which is more evident in women [24]. Social marginalization and employment discrimination are part of the stigma [25]. Being obese, or even just overweight, may represent an exclusion criterion in job interviews or applications. Unlike disabled people, considered "not guilty" for their condition, the obese subject is yielded responsible for his own condition and penalized at various levels in our society [26].

7.2.2 The Metabolic-Nutritional-Psychological Rehabilitation in the Treatment of Obesity

The basic assumptions and criteria related to the metabolic-nutritional-psychological rehabilitation (MNPR) have been acknowledged in a consensus document promoted by the SIO (Italian Society of Obesity) and the SISDCA (Italian Society for the Study of Eating Disorders) published in 2010.

The rehabilitative interventions aim at recovering *functional competence*, at *building a barrier against the functional regression, at modifying the natural history of chronic diseases* and at improving the patient's quality of life. The rehabilitation is "a process of problem solving and education during which the person is leaded to the best quality of life on the physical, functional, social and emotional level with the least possible restriction in his operating decisions" [27–30].

The MNRP goals can be summarized as follows:

A. Short term:
   (a) To obtain a fat mass loss that reduces risk factors and comorbidity level
   (b) To optimize the residual functional ability and the basic everyday/social life independence, in order to minimize disability
   (c) To correct the patient's behaviour with regard to nutrition and physical activity and possibly associated eating disorders (i.e. BED, NES)
B. Long term:
   (a) To maintain a correct lifestyle (appropriate energy and nutrient balance)
   (b) To perform regular physical activity at least 2 h/week, at low-medium intensity (50 % of maximum heart rate)
   (c) To maintain the fat mass loss obtained in the short-term intervention, in order to reduce the associated risk factors

7.2.3 The Metabolic-Nutritional-Psychological Rehabilitation in the Healthcare Network

The most recent guidelines [31–37] agree as for the need of *multiple settings* for the treatment of obesity, from the long-term outpatient management to intensive, semi-residential and residential rehabilitation.

The metabolic-nutritional-psychological rehabilitation of the obese subject within the healthcare network is provided, as stated by the Consensus SIO-SISDCA 2010 [38], by the following facilities:

(a) Semi-residential: *day hospital, day service, community centre* (diagnostic and therapeutic rehabilitation)
(b) Residential: *residential intensive rehabilitation (cod. 56) or psychiatric rehabilitation* and therapeutic-rehabilitative community

7.2.4 Evaluation of Obesity-Related Disability

During the multidimensional evaluation of obese subjects, besides the nutritional status, the cardiovascular and respiratory risk, the metabolic profile, the lifestyle (dietary behaviour and physical activity), the psychological status, the quality of life, the disability, the motor functions and the osteoarticular problems have to be assessed.

Disability [39–49] in daily functional activities (*activities of daily life, instrumental activities of daily life*) is widely represented in health-related quality of life questionnaires. Obesity is strongly related with articular pain and osteoarthrosis [50, 51], which are crucial factors for disability [52]. Furthermore, different studies have shown that the probability to maintain a healthy status decreases inversely to BMI [52, 53].

There is an increasing number of studies devoted to the difficulties that obese subjects endure in:

1. Home mobility, personal hygiene, dressing on and off [2, 54–57]
2. Domestic activities/jobs (i.e. getting up from couch, climbing a stool, taking objects from the ground) [58–61]
3. Outdoor activities (i.e. pick up and carrying grocery shopping, walking more than 100 m, queueing) [62, 63]
4. Working activities (i.e. early fatigue, postural pain, frequent absences, inability to perform some tasks) [62–67]

7.2.5 Rehabilitation Intervention

The presence of cardiovascular, respiratory, osteoarticular, endocrine-metabolic and psychosocial symptoms often associated with obesity impose a complex multidisciplinary therapeutic-rehabilitative approach.

The literature and the clinical practice agree on a general principle: the treatment of the obesity-related disability must encompass the therapy of the underlying pathology [68–70]. Disability and functional deficits are – on a perverse feedback – important risk factors for obesity and its progressive worsening [15]: the spiral "obesity-complications-disability- weight gain" generates high costs both on the healthcare and the social system. The obese subject resembles a prisoner of his own body, trapped inside a cage.

Optimal outcomes can be obtained in subjects previously informed about their conditions, who are more capable to manage mood, anxiety or stress fluctuations, after an integrated individual rehabilitation project, considering:

(a) A nutritional intervention aimed at:
 • Restoring correct durable eating behaviours (quality, quantity and rhythm) based on Mediterranean diet standards (www.piramideitaliana.it)
 • Obtaining at least a 10 % of weight loss through the reduction of fat mass while preserving lean body mass
(b) A motor/functional rehabilitation program (functional re-education, physical reconditioning, motor rehabilitation) aimed at:
 • Reactivating hypotonic and hypotrophic muscular structures due to inactivity
 • Recovering articular range of motion
 • Improving cardiocirculatory and respiratory performance
 • Increasing energy expenditure
 • Increasing lean body mass/fat mass ratio
(c) A short focused therapeutic education and psychotherapeutic interventions [71–74] aimed at:
 • Recognizing patient's real needs
 • Correcting the patient's false beliefs about food and physical activity
 • Improving not only the knowledge but also the patient's skills proceeding from "knowing" to "knowing how to do" and "knowing how to be"
 • Improving the relation between the body and its appearance
 • Increasing the sense of responsibility toward the disease and the therapeutic approach
 • Improving the compliance to the treatments (short motivational counselling, etc.)
(d) The rehabilitation nursing aimed at:
 • Improving patient's responses to chronic pathology, disability and lifestyle
 • Increasing environmental and social supports
 • Protecting and stimulating functional and relational abilities in order to improve adherence to rehabilitative activities and social welfare
 • Teaching the control of simple clinical parameters (glycaemia, blood pressure)

7.2.6 Intensive Metabolic-Nutritional-Psychological Rehabilitation

The intensity of the rehabilitative intervention has to be modulated according to the patient's severity of obesity and comorbidities, to the psychological status and to the quality of life level.

Intensive rehabilitation represents a key point in the healthcare network when:

(a) The severity of clinical and/or psychiatric comorbidities of obesity is high.
(b) The impact on disability and quality of life of the patient is severe.
(c) There are a large number of interventions to be carried out [27].
(d) Previous interventions with minor intensity (i.e. outpatient long-term management, days service, day hospital) didn't bring the expected results and the risk for patient's health increased.

Intensive rehabilitation aims at preventing acute episodes (secondary prevention) with obvious advantages for health and quality of life of the subject and both direct and indirect healthcare costs. Literature shows that interdisciplinary interventions can modify the obesity natural history, reducing the incidence of complications or postponing their appearance, with important advantages also under the economic aspects [75, 76].

7.2.7 Metabolic-Nutritional-Psychological Rehabilitation and Surgery (Bariatric or Plastic-Reconstructive)

The rehabilitative intervention can be useful also during severe obese patient's approach to bariatric or plastic reconstructive surgery and during the follow-up period with the aim of reducing the preoperative risks, allowing an adequate and effective adaptation to the new clinical and functional situation, reducing the risk of nutritional deficiencies, strengthening the patient's compliance and improving long-term results.

The plastic-reconstructive remodelling can play an important role for the progressive correction of focused lipodystrophy and of the outcomes of weight loss. In particular, cutaneous-adipose voluminous abscess removal and abdominal, crural and pubic dermolipectomy allow the reduction of functional difficulties and can foster motivation to continue the rehabilitation program. The interventions after significant weight loss (abdominoplasty, mastoplasty, mastopexy, brachioplasty, crural lifting) allow the correction of severe blemishes with potential positive effects on quality of life.

7.2.8   Metabolic-Nutritional-Psychological Rehabilitation Program

The metabolic-nutritional-psychological rehabilitation program has to be granted also in the absence of an acute episode based on the disability level and clinical appropriateness for rehabilitation care.

Disability: to be evaluated with specific scales for obesity aimed at assessing the impact on quality of life and considering in particular:

• Pain, stiffness and functional limitations
• Interaction skills with external environment
• Psychological and cognitive status
• ADL and IADL disability [16, 77–79]

Validated instruments like the Sickness Impact Profile (SIP) and the Nottingham Health Profile (NHP) cover only the basic everyday life activities and an elevated number of patients achieve the higher score (*ceiling effect*). The questionnaire SF-36 has different dimensions, but it is not obese specific, even if it shows sensitivity to the weight loss impact on *health-related quality of life* [80, 81], Therefore it provides overall information about function but not about specific disability problems related to obesity [54].

On the basis of literature and our experience, the SIO has proposed the Test SIO for the obesity-related disabilities (TSO-RD) as an instrument for the evaluation of the obesity-related disability. The questionnaire is composed by 7 sections, with 36 items exploring the following disability dimensions: pain, stiffness, ADL and house mobility, house activities, outdoor activities, working activities and social life (Fig. 7.1). The degree of disability is evaluated comparing the obtained score with the maximum score achievable on the scale (360 points). It is considered disabled a subject that yields an overall score over 33 % or with a score $\geq 8/10$ in one single item. The TSO-RD has been developed from a multicentric study that involved 16 Italian institutes. A significant relationship between the TSO-RD score and all the parameters considered (quality of life, muscular strength, articular resistance and mobility) was observed [82].

Appropriateness: the access to the rehabilitation *setting* must occur with an appropriate use of the resources of the healthcare system so that these will be adequate to the patient's clinical-functional needs. In line with the literature [30–32, 72, 83] and the experience from different working groups in Italy, SIO has proposed the *CASCO-R tool (Comprehensive Appropriateness Scale for the Care of Obesity in Rehabilitation)*. The sheet specifies the intensity of the intervention (from dietary and clinical nutrition outpatient facility to day service/day hospital and residential intensive rehabilitation) based on clinical parameters. The CASCO-R includes 4 sections: obesity degree and complications risk level; clinical, functional and metabolic comorbidities; risk factors that increase obesity-related morbidity; and previous rehabilitative hospitalizations (Fig. 7.2). The CASCO-R and its threshold values have been investigated in a multicentric study that has involved 449 Italian patients.

TSD•OC
SIO Obesity-Related Disability Test

Patient _____ date: _____

assessment admission O   discharge O

Pain

10 8 6 4 2 0
Pain when walking

10 8 6 4 2 0
Pain in going up the stairs

10 8 6 4 2 0
Night pain

10 8 6 4 2 0
Pain at rest

10 8 6 4 2 0
Pain when carrying weights

Score in pain section:_____/50

Stiffness

10 8 6 4 2 0
Stiffness at morning awakening

10 8 6 4 2 0
Stiffness during the day

Score in rigidity section:_____/20

Function and autonomy in daily life activities (ADL & mobility indoor)

10 8 6 4 2 0
Difficulty in using the bathroom

10 8 6 4 2 0
Difficulty in the personal hygiene (bidet, washing the back, getting in and out the bath)

10 8 6 4 2 0
Difficulty to get dressed (put on and off socks or stockings)

10 8 6 4 2 0
Difficulty in putting on and off the shoes or in lacing them

10 8 6 4 2 0
Difficulty in foot care and hygiene

Fig. 7.1 SIO Obesity-Related Disability Test (TSD•OC)

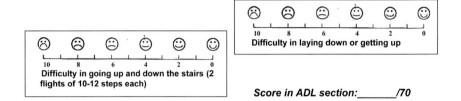

Score in ADL section:_____/70

Function and autonomy in housework

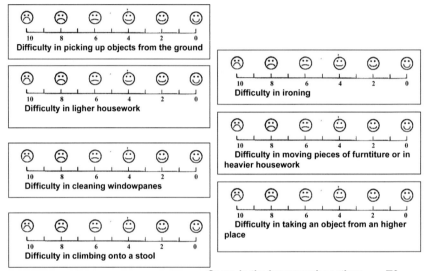

Score in the housework section:____/70

Function and autonomy in outdoor activities (IADL)

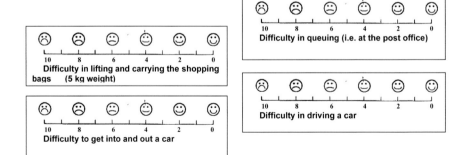

Fig 7.1 (continued)

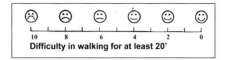

Difficulty in walking for at least 20'

Score in IADL section:_____/50

Function and autonomy at work (occupational activities)

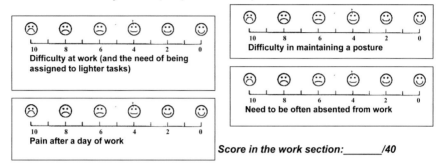

Score in the work section:_____/40

Function and autonomy in the social life

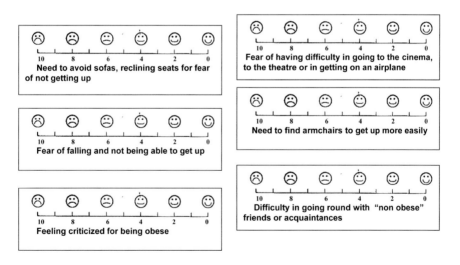

Score in social life section:_____/60

Fig 7.1 (continued)

	Pain	Stiffness	ADL	Housework	IADL	Work	Social life	Total	Ratio
Max score	50	20	70	70	50	40	60	360	>33%

In case the patient can't answer to some questions, specify the maximum score obtainable in each scale and relate the total score obtained to the maximum obtainable, summing up these new scale scores.

Maximum score obtained to any item of the dimension….	
Pain	
Siffness	
ADL	
Housework	
IADL	
Work	
Social life	

References

1. Bellamy N, Buchanan WW, Goldsmith CH, Campbell J, Stitt LW: Validation study of Womac: a health status instrument for measuring clinically important patient relevant outcomes to antirheumatic drug therapy in patients with osteoarthritis of the hip or knee. J Rheumatol 1988, 15, 1833-40
2. Ferraro KF, Su Y, Gretebeck RJ, Black DR, Badylak SF: Body mass index and disability in adulthood. Am J publ Health 2002, 92, 834-840
3. Guallar-Castillon P, Sagardui-Villamor J, Banegas JR, Graciani A, Schmid Fornes N, Lopez Garcia E, Rodriguez-Artalejo F: Waist circumference as a predictor of disability among older adults. Obesity 2007, 15, 233244
4. Han TS, Tijjhuis MAR, Lean MEJ, Seidell JC: Quality of life in relation to overweight and body fat distribution. Am J Publ Health 1998, 88, 1814-20
5. Heo M, Allison DB, Faith MS, Zhu S, Fontaine KR: Obesity and quality of life. Obes Res 2003, 11, 209-216
6. Houston DK, Stevens J, Cat J: Abdominal fat distribution and functional limitations and disability in a biracial cohort. Int J Obes 2005, 29, 1457-1463
7. Houston DK, Ding J, Nicklas BJ, Harris TB, Lee JS, Nevitt MC, Rubin SM, Tylavsky FA, Kritcevsky SB: The association between weight history and physical performance in the Health, Aging and Body Composition study. Int J Obes 2007, 1-8
8. Jenkins KR: Body-weight change and physical functioning among young old adults. J Ageing Health 2004, 16, 248-266
9. Kostka T, Bogus K: independent contribution of overweight/obesity and physical inactivity to lower health-related quality of life in community-dwelling older subjects. Z-Gerontol Geriatr 2007, 40, 43-51
10. Larrieu S, Peres K, Letenneur L, Berr C, Dartigues JF, Ritchie K, Fevrier B, Alperovitch A, Barberger-Gateau P: Relationship between BMI and different domains of disability in older persons. Int J Obes 2004, 28, 1555-60
11. Larsson UE, Mattson E: Preceived disability and observed functional limitations in obese women. Int J Obes 2001, 25, 1705-12Lean MEJ, Han TS, Seidell JC: Impairment of health and quality of life in people with large waist circumference. Lancet 1998, 351, 853-6
12. Lidstone JSM, Ells LJ, Finn P, Whittaker VJ, Wilkinson JR, Summerbell CD: Independent associations between weight status and disability in adults. Public Health 2006, 120, 412-7
13. Okoro CA, Hootman JM, Strine TW, Balluz LS, Mokdad AH: Disability, arthritis and body weight among adults 45 years and older. Obes Res 2004, 12, 854-861

CASCO-R
Comprehensive Appropriateness Scale for the Care of Obesity in Rehabilitation

Patient name			Date	
			Attribuable score	Obtained score
Obesity degree And related risk for cardiovascular and metabolic disorders		BMI ≥ 40 Kg/m²	8	
		BMI 35-39.9 Kg/m²	6	
		BMI 30-34.9 Kg/m²	4	
		Waist circumference > 102 cm ♂; 88 cm ♀	2	
Comorbidity	Dyslipidemia	LDL-cholesterol ≥ 130 mg/dl or antidyslipidemic medications	4	
		HDL-cholesterol ≤ 40 mg/dl ♂; 50 mg/dl ♀	2	
		Triglyceride > 150 mg/dl or antidyslipidemic medications	1	
	Impaired glucose metabolism	IFG (fasting blood glucose 110-125 mg/dl) or hyperinsulinemia [insulin > 25 mcU/ml or >80 mcU/ml on the 75-g OGTT between 60' and 120' or with a peak > 90') or HOMA (Glic * Ins/405) > 2.77	2	
		IGT (2 h glucose levels of 140 to 199 mg/dl on the 75-g OGTT)	4	
		T2DM (fasting plasma glucose ≥ 126 mg/dl or 2h glucose levesl ≥ 200 mg/dl on the 75-g OGTT) or antidiabetic medications	6	
	Cardiovascular system	Hypertension (SBP > 130 mmHg or DBP > 85 mmHg or antihypertensivemedications)	3	
		Atherosclerosis (ischemic cardiomiopathy, stroke, ...)	4	
		NYHA: class III (marked limitation in activity due to symptoms, even during less-than-ordinary activity) or IV (severe limitations; symptoms even while at rest)	4	
		Asymptomatic left ventricular hypertrophy	3	
	Respiratory system	OSAS, restrictive respiratory failure	4	
		Dyspnea, Epworth scale > 10	2	
	Skeletal system	Osteoarthritis (hip, knees, spine)	3	
	Genitourinary system	Gynecological problems (dysmenorrhea, PCOS)	2	
		Impaired sexual function	2	
		Urinary incontinence	2	
	Gastrointestinal tract	NAFLD, biliary calculi	1	
	Proinflammatory status	C-reactive protein > 10 mg/l	3	
	Procoagulant status	Fibrinogen > 450 mg/dl	3	
Risk facotors that contribute to increase the obeisty-related comorbidity	Family diseases	Early cardiovascular diseases (myocardial infarction, stroke, sudden death before age 65 in ♀ relatives or before age 55 in ♂ relatives)	4	
	Age	≥ 45 years ♂; 55 years ♀ (or premature menopause without hormonal replacement treatment)	2	
	Life habits	Sedentary lifestyle (<10 METs/week)	1	
		Smoking > 10 cigarettes/day	1	
	Behaviour	Psychic alterations (depression, anxiety)	2	
		Eating disorders: prandial hyperfagia, grazing, emotional eating, night eating	3	
		Eating disorders: bulimia nervosa, BED	4	
	Anamnesis	Failure of > 3 out-patient treatments for weight loss	2	
	Malnutrition (undernutrition)	Hb < 12 g/dl ♀, 13 g/dl ♂; albuminemia < 35 g/l; total cholesterol < 150 mg/dl (without antidyslipidemic medications); arm circumference < 22 cm; calf circumference < 31 cm	4	
Previous in-patient rehabilitation tretaments		First return (weight gain > 50% of that lost during the previous admission)	-5	
		Following returns (weight gain > 50% of that lost during the previous admission)	-10	
a. >25: in-patient rehabilitation b. 20-25: intensive out-patient rehabilitation c. < 20: out-patient treatment			TOT	

Fig. 7.2 Comprehensive Appropriateness Scale for the Care of Obesity in Rehabilitation (CASCO-R)

Validation was performed by comparing the CASCO-R score vs workload defined though ward medical and nurses interventions, diagnostic procedures and adverse clinical events [84–86]. Threshold values have been found for the correct allocation of patients in the different rehabilitative *settings*:

- >25: admission in residential intensive metabolic-nutritional psychological rehabilitation
- 20–25: admission in *day-hospital/day-service* intensive metabolic-nutritional psychological rehabilitation
- <20: specialistic outpatient setting

As previously pointed out by the SIO-SISDCA 2010 Consensus [38] also acute care interventions are part of the healthcare and rehabilitative network. A one-week hospitalization can precede the rehabilitative program or follow an acute event or it can be programmed according to the comorbidity level and clinical risk (CASCO-R ≥ 30). Acute care admission aims at stabilizing the clinical conditions and performing multidimensional evaluation for a successful rehabilitative program.

7.2.9 Intensive Rehabilitation Duration

Presently, the Italian laws regarding intensive rehabilitation for obese patients indicate that 60 days do represent a congruous period in order to obtain positive outcomes. However, this aspect is not acknowledged by all Italian regions. The post-acute rehabilitation hospital stay is generally limited to a maximum of 30 days which, in our opinion, is not adequate to fulfill the complex multidisciplinary needs of patients undergoing metabolic-nutritional-psychological rehabilitation.

Longitudinal studies are needed to estimate results in terms of costs and benefits [29].

References

1. Lean ME, Han TS, Seidell JC (1998) Impairment of health and quality of life in people with large waist circumference. Lancet 351(9106):853–856
2. Han TS, Tijhuis MA, Lean ME, Seidell JC (1998) Quality of life in relation to overweight and body fat distribution. Am J Public Health 88(12):1814–1820
3. Wannamethee SG, Shaper AG, Walker M (2005) Overweight and obesity and weight change in middle aged men: impact on cardiovascular disease and diabetes. J Epidemiol Community Health 59(2):134–139
4. Stucki A, Daansen P, Fuessl M, Cieza A, Huber E, Atkinson R et al (2004) ICF core set for obesity. J Rehabil Med 36(Suppl 44):107–113
5. Kim JY, Oh DJ, Yoon TY, Choi JM, Choe BK (2007) The impacts of obesity on psychological well-being: a cross-sectional study about depressive mood and quality of life. J Prev Med Public Health 40(2):191–195
6. Fontaine KR, Redden DT, Wang C, Westfall AO, Allison DB (2003) Years of life lost due to obesity. JAMA 289(2):187–193

7. Fontaine KR, Barofsky I, Bartlett SJ, Franckowiak SC, Andersen RE (2004) Weight loss and health-related quality of life: results at 1-year follow-up. Eat Behav 5(1):85–88
8. Janicke DM, Marciel KK, Ingerski LM, Novoa W, Lowry KW, Sallinen BJ et al (2007) Impact of psychosocial factors on quality of life in overweight youth. Obesity (Silver Spring) 15(7):1799–1807
9. Petroni ML, Villanova N, Avagnina S, Fusco MA, Fatati G, Compare A et al (2007) Psychological distress in morbid obesity in relation to weight history. Obes Surg 17(3):391–399
10. Hughes AR, Farewell K, Harris D, Reilly JJ (2007) Quality of life in a clinical sample of obese children. Int J Obes (Lond) 31(1):39–44
11. Sach TH, Barton GR, Doherty M, Muir KR, Jenkinson C, Avery AJ (2007) The relationship between body mass index and health-related quality of life: comparing the EQ-5D, EuroQol VAS and SF-6D. Int J Obes (Lond) 31(1):189–196
12. Chen EY, Bocchieri-Ricciardi LE, Munoz D, Fischer S, Katterman S, Roehrig M et al (2007) Depressed mood in class III obesity predicted by weight-related stigma. Obes Surg 17(5):669–671
13. Ashmore JA (2008) Weight-based stigmatization, psychological di stress, and binge eating behaviour among obese treatment-seeking adults. Eat Behav 9:203–209
14. Peytremann-Bridevaux I, Burnad B (2009) Inventory and perspectives of chronic disease management programs in Switzerland: an exploratory survey. Int J Integr Care 9:e93
15. Forhan M (2009) An analysis of disability models and the application of the ICF to obesity. Disabil Rehabil 31(16):1382–1388
16. Ferraro KF, Su YP, Gretebeck RJ, Black DR, Badylak SF (2002) Body mass index and disability in adulthood: a 20-year panel study. Am J Public Health 92(5):834–840
17. Kostka T, Bogus K (2007) Independent contribution of overweight/obesity and physical inactivity to lower health-related quality of life in community-dwelling older subjects. Z Gerontol Geriatr 40(1):43–51
18. Liou TH, Pi-Sunyer FX, Laferrere B (2005) Physical disability and obesity. Nutr Rev 63(10):321–331
19. Bliddal H, Christensen R (2006) The management of osteoarthritis in the obese patient: practical considerations and guidelines for therapy. Obes Rev 7(4):323–331
20. Kostka T, Praczko K (2007) Interrelationship between physical activity, symptomatology of upper respiratory tract infections, and depression in elderly people. Gerontology 53(4):187–193
21. Guallar-Castillon P, Sagardui-Villamor J, Banegas JR, Graciani A, Fornes NS, Lopez Garcia E et al (2007) Waist circumference as a predictor of disability among older adults. Obesity (Silver Spring) 15(1):233–244
22. Blaum CS, Xue QL, Michelon E, Semba RD, Fried LP (2005) The association between obesity and the frailty syndrome in older women: the Women's Health and Aging Study. J Am Geriatr Soc 53:927–934
23. Puhl RM, Brownell KD (2006) Confronting and coping with weight stigma: an investigation of overweight and obese adults. Obesity (Silver Spring) 14(10):1802–1815
24. Lim W, Thomas KS, Bardwell WA, Dimsdale JE (2008) Which measures of obesity are related to depressive symptoms and in whom? Psychosomatics 49(1):23–28
25. Falkner NH, French SA, Jeffery RW, Neumark-Sztainer D, Sherwood NE, Morton N (1999) Mistreatment due to weight: prevalence and sources of perceived mistreatment in women and men. Obes Res 7(6):572–576
26. Crandall CS (1994) Prejudice against fat people: ideology and self-interest. J Pers Soc Psychol 66(5):882–894
27. Linee Guida del Ministero della Sanità per le attività di Riabilitazione – GU 30 maggio (1998) 124
28. Ministero della Salute – Riabilitazione – Piano di indirizzo 6.10.2010

29. Towards a common language for function, disability and health ICF. Geneva: WHO 2002 (WHO/EIP/GPE/CAS/01.3)
30. International classification of functioning, disability and health (ICF) (2007) WHO
31. National Institutes of Health (1998) Clinical guidelines on the identification, evaluation and treatment of overweight and obesity in adults. The evidence report. Obes Res 6(Suppl 2):51S–209S
32. Wadden T, Stunkard A (eds) (2002) Handbook of obesity treatment. Guilford, New York
33. Fairburn C, Brownell K (eds) (2002) Eating disorders and obesity. A comprehensive handbook, 2nd edn. Guilford, New York
34. Wilson GT, Shafran R (2005) Eating disorders guidelines from NICE. Lancet 365(9453):79–81
35. Birmingham CL, Jones P, Hoffer LJ (2003) The management of adult obesity. Eat Weight Disord 8(2):157–163
36. Lau DC, Douketis JD, Morrison KM, Hramiak IM, Sharma AM, Ur E (2007) 2006 Canadian clinical practice guidelines on the management and prevention of obesity in adults and children. CMAJ 176(8):S1–S13
37. Basdevant A, Guy-Grand B (eds) (2004) Médecine de l'obésité. Flammarion, Paris
38. Donini LM, Cuzzolaro M, Spera G, Badiali M, Basso N, Bollea MR, Bosello O, Brunani A, Busetto L, Cairella G, Cannella C, Capodaglio P, Carbonelli MG, Castellaneta E, Castra R, Clini E, Contaldo F, Dalla Ragione L, Dalle Grave R, D'Andrea F, Del Balzo V, De Cristofaro P, Di Flaviano E, Fassino S, Ferro AM, Forestieri P, Franzoni E, Gentile MG, Giustini A, Jacoangeli F, Lubrano C, Lucchin L, Manara F, Marangi G, Marcelli M, Marchesini G, Marri G, Marrocco W, Melchionda N, Mezzani B, Migliaccio P, Muratori F, Nizzoli U, Ostuzzi R, Panzolato G, Pasanisi F, Persichetti P, Petroni ML, Pontieri V, Prosperi E, Renna C, Rovera G, Santini F, Saraceni V, Savina C, Scuderi N, Silecchia G, Strollo F, Todisco P, Tubili C, Ugolini G, Zamboni M (2010) Obesità e disturbi dell'Alimentazione. Indicazioni per i diversi livelli di trattamento. Documento di Consensus. Eat Weight Disord 15(1–2 Suppl):1–31
39. Lidstone JS, Ells LJ, Finn P, Whittaker VJ, Wilkinson JR, Summerbell CD (2006) Independent associations between weight status and disability in adults: results from the Health Survey for England. Public Health 120(5):412–417
40. Evers Larsson U, Mattsson E (2001) Functional limitations linked to high body mass index, age and current pain in obese women. Int J Obes Relat Metab Disord 25(6):893–899
41. Ostbye T, Dement JM, Krause KM (2007) Obesity and workers' compensation: results from the Duke Health and Safety Surveillance System. Arch Intern Med 167(8):766–773
42. Karnehed N, Rasmussen F, Kark M (2007) Obesity in young adulthood and later disability pension: a population-based cohort study of 366,929 Swedish men. Scand J Public Health 35(1):48–54
43. Banegas JR, Lopez-Garcia E, Graciani A, Guallar-Castillon P, Gutierrez-Fisac JL, Alonso J et al (2007) Relationship between obesity, hypertension and diabetes, and health-related quality of life among the elderly. Eur J Cardiovasc Prev Rehabil 14(3):456–462
44. Gunstad J, Luyster F, Hughes J, Waechter D, Rosneck J, Josephson R (2007) The effects of obesity on functional work capacity and quality of life in phase II cardiac rehabilitation. Prev Cardiol 10(2):64–67
45. Williams J, Wake M, Hesketh K, Maher E, Waters E (2005) Health-related quality of life of overweight and obese children. JAMA 293(1):70–76
46. Ells LJ, Lang R, Shield JP, Wilkinson JR, Lidstone JS, Coulton S et al (2006) Obesity and disability – a short review. Obes Rev 7(4):341–345
47. Peeters A, Bonneux L, Nusselder WJ, De Laet C, Barendregt JJ (2004) Adult obesity and the burden of disability throughout life. Obes Res 12(7):1145–1151
48. Jenkins KR (2004) Obesity's effects on the onset of functional impairment among older adults. Gerontologist 44(2):206–216
49. Visser M, Kritchevsky SB, Goodpaster BH, Newman AB, Nevitt M, Stamm E et al (2002) Leg muscle mass and composition in relation to lower extremity performance in men and women

aged 70 to 79: the health, aging and body composition study. J Am Geriatr Soc 50(5):897–904

50. Hartz AJ, Fischer ME, Bril G, Kelber S (1986) The association of obesity with jointy pain and ostheoarthritis in the HANES data. J Chron Dis 39:311–319

51. Anandacoomarasamy A, Fransen M, March L (2009) Systemic disorders with rheumatic manifestations. Curr Opin Rheumatol 21(1):71–77

52. Visser M, Langlois J, Guralnik JM et al (1998) High body fatness, but no low fat-free mass, predicts disability in older men and women: the Cardiovascular Health Study. Am J Clin Nutr 68:584–590

53. Rejeski WJ (2008) Obesity influences transitional states of disability in older adults with knee pain. Arch Phys Med Rehabil 89:2102–2107

54. Wearing SC, Hennig EM, Byrne NM, Steele JR, Hills AP (2006) The biomechanics of restricted movement in adult obesity. Obes Rev 7(1):13–24

55. Larsson UE, Mattsson E (2001) Perceived disability and observed functional limitations in obese women. Int J Obes (Lond) 25:1705–1712

56. Holm K, Li S, Spector N, Hicks F, Carlson E, Lanuza D (2001) Obesity in adult and children: a call for action. J Adv Nurs 36:266–269

57. Lamb SE, Guralnik JM, Buchner DM et al (2000) Factors that modify the association between knee pain and mobility limitation in older women: the Women's Health and Aging Study. Ann Rheum Dis 59:331–337

58. Spyropoulos P, Pisciotta JC, Pavlou KN, Cairns MA, Simon SR (1991) Biomechanical Gait Analysis in obese men. Arch Phys Med Rehabil 72:1065–1070

59. Vismara L et al (2007) Clinical implications of gait analysis in the rehabilitation of adult patients with Prader-Willi Syndrome: a cross-sectional comparative study. J Neuroeng Rehabil 4:14. doi:10.1186/1743-0003-4-14

60. Xu X, Mirka GA, Hsiang SM (2008) The effects of obesity on lifting performance. Appl Ergon 39(1):93–98

61. Larsson EU, Mattsson E (2001) Functional limitations linked to high body mass index, age and current pain in obese women. Int J Obes Relat Metab Disord 25(6):893–899

62. Finkelstein EA, Chen H, Prabhu M, Trogdon JG, Corso PS (2007) The relationship between obesity and injuries among U.S. adults. Am J Health Promot 21(5):460–468

63. Tunceli K, Li K, Williams LK (2006) Long-term effects of obesity on employment and work limitations among U.S. Adults, 1986 to 1999. Obesity (Silver Spring) 14(9):1637–1646

64. Schmier JK, Jones ML, Halpern MT (2006) Cost of obesity in the workplace. Scand J Work Environ Health 32(1):5–11

65. Thompson DL (2007) The costs of obesity: what occupational health nurses need to know. AAOHN J 55(7):265–270

66. Coggon D, Croft P, Kellingray S, Barrett D, McLaren M, Cooper C (2000) Occupational physical activities and osteoarthritis of the knee. Arthritis Rheum 43(7):1443–1449

67. Werner RA, Franzblau A, Albers JW, Armstrong TJ (1997) Influence of body mass index and work activity on the prevalence of median mononeuropathy at the wrist. Occup Environ Med 54(4):268–271

68. Coggon D, Reading I, Croft P, McLaren M, Barrett D, Cooper C (2001) Knee osteoarthritis and obesity. Int J Obes Relat Metab Disord 25(5):622–627

69. Tchernof A, Nolan A, Sites CK, Ades PA, Poehlman ET (2002) Weight loss reduces C-reactive protein levels in obese postmenopausal women. Circulation 105(5):564–569

70. Giugliano D, Ceriello A, Esposito K (2006) The effects of diet on inflammation: emphasis on the metabolic syndrome. J Am Coll Cardiol 48(4):677–685

71. Avenell A, Sattar N, Lean M (2006) ABC of obesity. Management: Part I – behaviour change, diet, and activity. BMJ 333(7571):740–743

72. Lang A, Froelicher ES (2006) Management of overweight and obesity in adults: behavioral intervention for long-term weight loss and maintenance. Eur J Cardiovasc Nurs 5(2):102–114

73. Sarsan A, Ardic F, Ozgen M, Topuz O, Sermez Y (2006) The effects of aerobic and resistance exercises in obese women. Clin Rehabil 20(9):773–782
74. National Heart Lung and Blood Institute (NHLBI), North American Association for the Study of Obesity (NAASO) (2000) Practical Guide to the identification, evaluation and treatment of overweight and obesity in adults. National Institutes of Health, Bethesda
75. Wolf AM, Siadaty M, Yaeger B, Conaway MR, Crowther JQ, Nadler JL, Bovbjerg VE (2007) Effects of lifestyle intervention on health care costs: Improving Control with Activity and Nutrition (ICAN). J Am Diet Assoc 107(8):1365–1373
76. Allender S, Rayner M (2007) The burden of overweight and obesity-related ill health in the UK. Obes Rev 8(5):467–473
77. Houston DK, Stevens J, Cai J, Morey MC (2005) Role of weight history on functional limitations and disability in late adulthood: the ARIC study. Obes Res 13(10):1793–1802
78. Larrieu S, Peres K, Letenneur L, Berr C, Dartigues JF, Ritchie K et al (2004) Relationship between body mass index and different domains of disability in older persons: the 3C study. Int J Obes Relat Metab Disord 28(12):1555–1560
79. Houston DK, Ding J, Nicklas BJ, Harris TB, Lee JS, Nevitt MC et al (2007) The association between weight history and physical performance in the Health, Aging and Body Composition study. Int J Obes (Lond) 31(11):1680–1687
80. Choban PS, Onyejekwe J, Burge JC, Flancbaum L (1999) A health status assessment of impact of weight loss following Rox-en-Y gastric bypass for clinically severe obesity. J Am Coll Surg 188:491–497
81. Fontaine KR, Barofsky I, Andersen RE, Bartlett SJ, Wiersema L, Cheskin LJ, Franckowiak SC (1999) Impact of weight loss on health-related quality of life. Qual Life Res 8:275–277
82. Donini LM, Brunani A, Sirtori A, Savina C, Tempera S, Cuzzolaro M, Spera G, Cimolin V, Precilios H, Raggi A, Capodaglio P (2011) Assessing disability in morbidly obese individuals: the Italian Society of Obesity test for obesity-related disabilities. Disabil Rehabil 33(25–26):2509–2518
83. Bray GA, Bellanger T (2006) Epidemiology, trends, and morbidities of obesity and the metabolic syndrome. Endocrine 29(1):109–117
84. Donini LM, Dalle Grave R, Di Flaviano E, Gentile MG, Mezzani B, Pandolfo Mayme M, Brunani A, Rovera G, Santini F, Lenzi A, Cuzzolaro M (2014) Assessing the appropriateness of the level of care for morbidly obese subjects: validation of the CASCO-R scale. Ann Ig 26(3):195–204. doi:10.7416/ai.2014.1977
85. Pandolfo M, Savina C, Tempera S, Donini LM, Cuzzolaro M, Spera G, del Balzo V, Petroni ML, Brunani A (2010) SIO-SISDCA Task Force: SIO Clinical Appropriateness chart (SSA-RMNP-O) for the metabolic, nutritional and psychologicaln rehabilitation of obesity Atti XII International Conference on Obesity – ICO 2010 – Stockholm, 11–15 July 2010
86. Corsi R, Pandolfo MM, Tempera S, Savina C, Donini LM, Cuzzolaro M, Spera G, del Balzo V, Petroni ML, Brunani A (2010) ed il gruppo di lavoro SIO-SISDCA: Appropriatezza ad un percorso di riabilitazione metabolico psico nutrizionale per i soggetti obesi. Atti Congr Naz ANMDO – Napoli 19–22 maggio 2010, p 33

Part IV

Obesity in Particular Conditions and Treatment Algorithm

Eating Disorders and Obesity

8

Massimo Cuzzolaro

8.1 Classification and Diagnosis

Recommendations

Treatment and care of patients with obesity require assessment of eating behavior to identify possible eating disorders. (*Level of evidence VI, Strength of recommendation A*)

In DSM-5 (*Diagnostic and Statistical Manual of Mental Disorders*, Fifth Edition), the "Feeding and eating disorders" section provides diagnostic criteria for pica, rumination disorder, avoidant/restrictive food intake disorder, anorexia nervosa, bulimia nervosa, binge eating disorder, other specified feeding or eating disorder, and unspecified feeding or eating disorder.

In particular, binge eating disorder (BED) is generally associated with obesity. To identify BED and other disordered eating patterns is a necessary step for both medical and surgical treatments of obesity. (*Level of evidence III, Strength of recommendation A*)

Individuals with BED-obesity present higher psychiatric comorbidity than individuals with non-BED-obesity and require psychological/psychiatric evaluation. (*Level of evidence III, Strength of recommendation A*)

Bulimia nervosa and some other disordered eating behaviors that do not appear in DSM-5 as specific diagnostic categories may be associated with

Massimo Cuzzolaro, Former researcher and professor of psychiatry – University of Roma Sapienza
Eating and Weight Disorders. Studies on Anorexia Bulimia Obesity – Editor-in-Chief

M. Cuzzolaro
Eating and Weight Disorders, Editor-in-Chief, Sapienza University of Roma, Former Researcher and Professor of Psychiatry, Via Fedi 12, Campiglia Marittima, LI 57021, Italy
e-mail: massimo.cuzzolaro@alice.it; massimo.cuzzolaro@gmail.com

© Springer International Publishing Switzerland 2016
P. Sbraccia et al. (eds.), *Clinical Management of Overweight and Obesity: Recommendations of the Italian Society of Obesity (SIO)*,
DOI 10.1007/978-3-319-24532-4_8

overweight and obesity: problematic restriction, hyperphagia, selective food craving (sweet, sweetened beverages, chocolate, etc.), grazing, emotional eating, night eating. They require clinical attention. (*Level of evidence VI, Strength of recommendation A*)

Self-report questionnaires and semi-structured diagnostic interviews can be helpful before, during, and after treatment to evaluate attitudes and behaviors, changes, and outcome. (*Level of evidence III, Strength of recommendation B*)

Table 8.1 goes over the main points of DSM-5 diagnostic criteria [1] for bulimia nervosa (BN) and binge eating disorder (BED). Atypical or subthreshold clinical pictures (low frequency or short duration BN or BED) are included in the DSM-5 diagnostic category of other specified feeding or eating disorder (OSFED).

In DSM-5, night eating syndrome (NES) is not an autonomous diagnostic category. It is included in the abovementioned diagnostic category OSFED. Table 8.2 summarizes the consensus diagnostic criteria for NES that were proposed in 2010 by an international research group [2].

Table 8.1 DSM-5 diagnostic criteria for bulimia nervosa (BN) and binge eating disorder (BED) [1]

Clinical features	Bulimia nervosa	Binge eating disorder
Overweight/obesity	Not required; it may occur	Not required but it usually occurs
Regular (on average, at least weekly) binge eating for at least three months	Required	Required with distress regarding binge eating and at least three out of five descriptors (eating very rapidly, until feeling uncomfortably full, when not feeling hungry, alone, and/or feeling disgusted after overeating)
Regular (on average, at least weekly) compensatory behaviors: e.g., self-induced vomiting, laxatives and/or diuretics misuse, excessive exercise, fasting, etc.	Required	Do not occur or are occasional
Overvaluation of body weight and shape	Required	Not required but body image uneasiness usually occurs
Subtypes	None	None
Remission specifier	Full remission/partial remission	Full remission/partial remission
Severity specifier	Frequency of compensatory behaviors (*mild* 1–3/week, *moderate* 4–7, *severe* 8–13, *extreme* ≥14)	Frequency of binge eating episodes (*mild* 1–3/week, *moderate* 4–7, *severe* 8–13, *extreme* ≥14)

Table 8.2 Night eating syndrome (NES) [2]

Consumption of at least 25 % of daily caloric intake after the evening meal
and/or
Nocturnal awakenings with ingestions at least twice per week
Awareness of the eating episodes
Distress or impairment in functioning
The above criteria must be met for a minimum duration of 3 months

Comment

Current taxonomies [1, 3] classify eating disorders (ED) as psychiatric problems and obesity as a general medical condition. However, connections and overlaps between the two fields are so relevant that it is not groundless to keep talking about them as two sides of the same coin and to use wide-ranging expressions like nonhomeostatic eating disorders or weight-related disorders [4–8].

Genetic predisposition to obesity was found in individuals with bulimia nervosa (BN) [9]. Overweight is a risk factor for bulimia nervosa (BN) [10], and increasing numbers of individuals with BN are also obese [11–15]. As regards anorexia nervosa, adolescents with a history of overweight/obesity represent a considerable portion of patients with restrictive ED [16]. Emerging research on anorexia nervosa (AN), bulimia nervosa (BN), and binge eating disorder (BED) suggests the importance of so-called *weight suppression* (the difference between highest past weight and current weight) as ED outcome predictor [17–20]. On the other hand, dieting and weight suppression may be risk factors for future increases in adiposity [21, 22]. To finish serious ED may appear after bariatric surgery. Segal and coworkers proposed a new category named *Post-Surgical Eating Avoidance Disorder* [23]. It is likely that such postoperative symptoms are underreported [24]. A large matched (2010 bariatric patients and 1916 controls) nonrandomized prospective intervention trial of the Swedish Obese Subjects (SOS) study found that higher tendency to eat in response to various internal and external cues shortly after bariatric surgery predicted less successful short- and long-term weight outcomes. Therefore, postoperative susceptibility for uncontrolled eating could be an important indicator of targeted interventions [25].

An episode of overeating with loss of control is called *binge eating*, a symptom that crosses the entire field of ED and the whole spectrum of body weights [26, 27]. Both observational and experimental studies focused on three possible risk factors for binge eating: deficits in emotion regulation processes [28, 29], unbalanced nutrition style (in particular, so-called problematic restriction) [30], and body dissatisfaction [31, 32]. In a recent research, structural equation modeling revealed that overvaluation of weight and shape and body dissatisfaction caused dietary restraint, thus triggering binge eating [31].

Binge eating disorder (BED) is an expression that indicates a particular syndrome usually associated with obesity. The core feature of BED is the presence of recurrent episodes of overeating with loss of control (like BN) and no regular use of inappropriate weight loss behaviors (unlike BN).

As regards ED, the most impactful change in DSM-5 was the official recognition of BED as a specific diagnostic category [1]. The frequency cut-point for DSM-5 diagnosis of BED is once per week for 3 months. BED is usually associated with obesity, and beginning from the last decade of the twentieth century [33] research on BED has firmly connected the psychiatric field of eating disorders with the medical area of obesity. This bridge has attracted increasing attention to the psychological and psychiatric aspects of obesity and contributed to the development of a multidimensional/multidisciplinary team approach for patients with eating and weight disorders [34].

Many studies and systematic reviews support the distinction between BED- and non-BED-obesity on the basis of different variables, in particular psychiatric comorbidity [28, 35–42], also using DSM-5 broader criteria [39, 43]. A recent survey found that mood and substance use disorders co-occur frequently among patients with BED [44]. In obesity surgery candidates, BED is associated with an increased prevalence of current and lifetime mood and anxiety disorders, beyond the already elevated rate observed with obesity class III [45]. Personality disorders are more frequent in obese patients with BED as well, in particular borderline, avoidant, and obsessive-compulsive personality pathology [44, 46, 47]. Health-related quality of life (HRQoL) is more damaged, especially mental HRQoL [48, 49]. A recent systematic review found that BED is also related to increased healthcare utilization and healthcare costs [49].

DSM-5 does not require overvaluation of body weight and shape for diagnosis, but body image uneasiness usually occurs in individuals with BED. A matched study verified that both men and women with BED-obesity suffer from a more negative body image [50]. Furthermore, a recent community survey found that body image disparagement could be a specifier for BED able to provide stronger information about severity than the DSM-5 rating based on binge eating frequency (see Table 8.1) [51].

However a question remains: does BED represent a really separate, reliable, and valid diagnostic category? For example Stunkard – who originally described binge eating associated with obesity [52] – proposed with Allison that the presence or absence of BED is not a useful distinction in selecting treatment for obese individuals and BED may be more useful as a marker of psychopathology than as a new distinct diagnostic entity [53]. A recent review concludes that, despite its inclusion in DSM-5 as an autonomous category, BED diagnosis and treatment strategies require further deepening [54].

Epidemiological studies on BED suffer from many limitations, and results are often discordant. Furthermore, DSM-5 formal diagnostic criteria are very recent [1]. However, in the United States BED seems to be the most common eating disorder. The results of the National Comorbidity Survey Replication, a face-to-face household study conducted in a large representative sample of adults ($n = 9282$) using the DSM-IV provisional criteria [55], indicated the following lifetime community prevalence rates: 3.5 % in women and 2.0 % in men; F to M ratio was 1.75:1.0. Furthermore, lifetime BED was significantly associated with current obesity class III (BMI $\geq$40 kg/m^2) [56]. A longitudinal study of 496 girls, using the new broader DSM-5 criteria, found that lifetime prevalence of BED by age 20 was 3.0 % and diagnostic crossover from BED to BN was very great [57]. An Italian three-phase community-based study evaluated 2,355 subjects aged >14 years and found an over-all lifetime prevalence of BED (DSM-IV provisional criteria) considerably lower than the American rates: 0.32 % [58]. The prevalence rates for BED (DSM-IV provisional criteria) appear particularly high among bariatric surgery candidates in many investigations [59, 60]. A large (2266 participants) multicenter study confirmed that a substantial proportion of bariatric surgery candidates report problematic eating behaviors (loss of control eating 43.4 %, night eating syndrome 17.7 %; binge eating disorder 15.7 %, bulimia nervosa 2 %) [61]. In a recent survey, an additional 3.43 % of bariatric surgery candidates met the diagnostic threshold for BED when using the new broader DSM-5 criteria in comparison with the old DSM-IV provisional criteria [43].

As well as BED and BN, a number of disordered eating behaviors may be associated with obesity, but definitions are often inconsistent [62].

- The term *hyperphagia* indicates habitual consumption of much more food than necessary without a subjective feeling of loss of control, unlike binge eating. Hyperphagia may contribute to obesity as observed in the general population and is a core symptom of some genetic disorders (e.g., Prader-Willi syndrome) [63]. In Prader-Willi syndrome, it seems unlikely that ghrelin levels are directly responsible for the switch to overeating because they are elevated long before the onset of hyperphagia that usually begins between the age of 2 and 8 [64].
- According to a recent review [65] (page 973), *grazing* (*picking*, *nibbling*) may be defined "as an eating behavior characterized by the repetitive eating … of small/modest amounts of food in an unplanned manner." Two subtypes – compulsive and noncompulsive grazing – can be distinguished on the basis of loss of control. Grazing is frequently associated with anorexia nervosa, bulimia nervosa, BED- and non-BED-obesity [66]. It is a significant predictor of weight regain after weight loss treatments and bariatric surgery [62, 67–70]. Mindfulness-based interventions can be helpful [71].
- A significant proportion of individuals with obesity report eating for emotional reasons (*emotional eating*). Emotional eating seems to be positively associated with general and eating psychopathology, binge eating, and negatively associated with mindfulness and body image flexibility [72]. An experimental study found that *high emotional eaters* ate significantly more after negative emotions (e.g., sad mood) than after positive emotions (e.g., joy mood) [73]. Experimental data [74] and a literature review [75] suggest that ghrelin, an eating-related gut-brain peptide, is involved in stress and reward-oriented behaviors and regulates anxiety and mood.
- Several studies have investigated *selective food craving* defined as an intense desire to consume a particular food or a specific food class that is difficult to resist (e.g., fats, carbohydrates, chocolate, sweets, etc.) [76, 77]. In recent years, the concept of food craving and the food addiction model seem to be relevant to eating and weight disorder treatment and prevention [78–84]. In a racially diverse sample of patients with BED-obesity, a recent survey found that a considerable subset (41.5 %) met the Yale Food Addiction Scale (YFAS) cutoff [85]. The strong reinforcing effects of both food and drugs are mediated by rapid dopamine increases in the brain reward circuitries that, in vulnerable individuals,

can override the brain's homeostatic control mechanisms [86]. A functional magnetic resonance imaging study examined the neural correlates of addictive-like eating behavior. High YFAS scores [87] were associated with comparable patterns of neural activation as substance dependence: elevated activation in reward circuitry (dorsolateral prefrontal cortex and caudate) in response to food cues (anticipated receipt) and reduced activation of inhibitory regions (lateral orbitofrontal cortex) in response to food intake (receipt) [88].

- In 2010, an international research group proposed a set of diagnostic criteria for the *night eating syndrome* (NES) [2] that, however, is not yet a DSM-5 diagnostic category [1]. Night eating behavior is frequent among people with obesity, particularly among bariatric surgery candidates [61, 89, 90].

A very large number of semi-structured interviews and self-report questionnaires are psychometrically sound and may be helpful to evaluate ED and body image disturbance and their changes over time. Six examples are the interview *Eating Disorder Examination*, EDE [91], and the questionnaires *Binge Eating Scale*, BES [92]; *Body Uneasiness Test*, BUT [93, 94]; *Questionnaire on Eating and Weight Patterns-5*, QEWP-5 [95]; SCOFF [96], and *Yale Food Addiction Scale*, YFAS [87, 97].

8.2 Treatment

Recommendations

Identification, assessment, and management of eating disorders and disordered eating behaviors are essential components of obesity treatment according to a multidimensional, multidisciplinary, and multiprofessional model. A multidisciplinary team is a group composed of members who should communicate on a regular basis about the shared clinical decision making. (*Level of evidence VI, Strength of recommendation A*)

Clinical assessment of patients with obesity and binge eating disorder (BED) or other disordered eating behaviors should take account of somatic conditions, obesity-related diseases, psycho-social problems, and psychiatric comorbidity. (*Level of evidence III, Strength of recommendation A*)

In most cases, ambulatory care provided on an outpatient basis is the recommended healthcare setting. Residential (hospitals, residential rehabilitative facilities) or semi-residential care (day-hospitals, day-care centers) may be necessary when obesity grade, eating disorder symptoms, medical and psychiatric comorbidity are very serious, risky, and outpatient treatment refractory. (*Level of evidence V, Strength of recommendation A*)

First-line treatment for bulimia nervosa and binge eating disorder in adults is psychological therapy, and there is an evidence base for individual cognitive behavior therapy (CBT), interpersonal therapy, dialectical behavior therapy. Self-help CBT and guided self-help CBT can be useful. There is small evidence for guided self-help CBT via telemedicine and the Internet as well. (*Level of evidence I, Strength of recommendation A*)

Lisdexamfetamine is the first medication that is FDA approved in the United States for BED. High dose fluoxetine (60 mg/day), other SSRI (selective serotonin reuptake inhibitors), many tricyclic antidepressants, and topiramate are effective for both bulimia nervosa and binge eating disorder. (*Level of evidence I, Strength of recommendation A*)

Pharmacotherapy may be an adjunctive treatment when people with obesity and eating disorders have limited response to psychotherapy alone or they present other psychiatric symptoms such as mood or anxiety disorders. (*Level of evidence I, Strength of recommendation A*)

Adverse effects of medications must be carefully monitored. (*Level of evidence I, Strength of recommendation A*)

Topiramate and/or orlistat may aid short-term weight loss. (*Level of evidence I, Strength of recommendation A*)

Weight loss management strategies are required to treat coexistent obesity. (*Level of evidence I, Strength of recommendation A*)

Preoperative eating disorders may have a negative effect on bariatric surgery outcome. BED does not represent an absolute contraindication to obesity surgery. However, pre- and postoperative assessment and treatment are required to maximize weight loss and general positive outcome. (*Level of evidence III, Strength of recommendation A*)

Eating disorders can develop after bariatric surgery. Postoperative assessment and treatment are required. (*Level of evidence V, Strength of recommendation A*)

Limited evidence suggests that some drugs (e.g., SSRI, melatonergic medications, topiramate), light therapy, and psychological interventions may be useful to treat *night eating syndrome* (NES). (*Level of evidence VI, Strength of recommendation B*)

A lifestyle intervention, tailored for individuals with serious psychiatric disorders taking psychotropic medications that usually induce weight gain, can reduce weight and improve fasting glucose levels. (*Level of evidence II, Strength of recommendation A*)

Table 8.3 makes a list of 23 studies on drug treatment of BED. It is inspired by a 2013 review article [121] modified and updated.

Comment

To evaluate signs and symptoms of ED is a necessary step so as to design a comprehensive [122] treatment plan for a patient with obesity [35, 123, 124] and to follow bariatric patients pre- and postsurgery [125–129]. Conversely, most patients with BED and increasing numbers with BN suffer also from obesity with current medical complications and obesity-related health risk [130]; as a consequence, they require medical assessment and may benefit from weight loss strategies [15, 54, 61]. In the last decades, almost all consensus documents and practice guidelines for the treatment of ED and obesity have recommended a multidimensional/multidisciplinary

Table 8.3 Drug treatment of BED: randomized controlled trials (RCT) and open-label[1] studies

Class	Drug	Binge eating	Weight loss
Tricyclic antidepressants (TCAs)	Imipramine [98]	a	
	Desipramine [99]	a	
Selective serotonin reuptake inhibitors (SSRIs)	Citalopram [100]	a	a
	S-citalopram [101]	a	a
	Fluoxetine [102]	a	a
	Fluvoxamine [103] [104]	a	a
	Sertraline [105]	a	a
Serotonin and/or norepinephrine reuptake inhibitors	Atomoxetine [106]	a	a
	Venlafaxine [107][1]	a	a
	Duloxetine [108]	a	a
Orlistat	Orlistat [109]		a
Antiepileptics	Topiramate [110–112] [113][1]	a	a
	Zonisamide [114] [115][1]	a	a
	Lamotrigine [116]		?
Other drugs	Baclofen [117]	a	
	Sodium oxybate [118] [1]	a	a
	Acamprosate [119]	?	?
	Lisdexanfetamine [120]	a	a

[a]Significant reduction of binge eating frequency or body weight in comparison with placebo
[1]Open-label trials

approach but, with a few exceptions [131], the guidelines for the assessment and treatment of obesity have devoted a scanty space to ED [13, 132, 133] and vice versa [134–136].

Several literature reviews have discussed the effects of individual and group psychological treatments for ED associated with obesity, in full, self-help and guided self-help forms, including web or Internet-based interventions [137–144]. Interpersonal psychotherapy (IPT) [145–148], cognitive behavioral therapy (CBT) [91, 149, 150], short-term cognitive behavioral therapy (CBT-st) [151], transdiagnostic cognitive behavioral therapy enhanced (CBT-E) [91, 152], mindfulness-based interventions [139, 153], dialectical behavior therapy (DBT) [154] can reduce binge eating frequency, but weight loss is usually modest and the long-term efficacy for the core and related symptoms of BED remains largely unknown. CBT and IPT appear to be the best supported psychotherapies for BN, whereas CBT seems to be the preferred psychological treatment for BED. However, a recent meta-analysis – which both examined direct comparisons between psychological treatments for BN and BED and considered the role of moderating variables – found that there is little support for diagnosis-based treatment specificity in psychological interventions for these two disorders [142].

A randomized controlled trial (RCT) found that group IPT is a feasible alternative to group CBT for the treatment of overweight patients with BED [146]. DBT [154] and group DBT [155] produced significant results in two RCTs. As to self-help, a randomized active-treatment concurrent control efficacy trial indicated that IPT and guided self-help based on cognitive behavior therapy (CBTgsh) were significantly more effective than behavioral weight loss treatment (BWL) in eliminating binge eating after 2 years [148]. Also, guided self-help based on dialectical behavior therapy (DBTgsh) produced significant short-term improvement in BED symptoms [156].

There are no evidence-based psychosocial treatments for adolescents with BN or BED associated with obesity but family treatment-behavior (FT-B) and supportive individual therapy could be helpful [141].

With reference to dropouts, a systematic literature review with metaregression analyses [140] revealed that manualized self-help interventions (bibliotherapy, CD-ROM, Internet-based intervention) may have a place in the treatment of BN and BED but dropout rates are usually very high. However, specialist guidance (*guided self-help*) can lead to higher intervention completion.

In conclusion, in a stepped-care treatment model CBTgsh should be a first-line treatment option for most patients with BED, with IPT or full CBT/CBT-E used for patients with high specific and/or general psychopathology.

Rapid response (defined as ≥ 65 % reduction in binge eating by week 4) seems to have important clinical implications for stepped-care treatment models for BED. An RCT found that, in rapid responders to group DBT, binge eating abstinence was significantly higher at the end of treatment and 1-year follow-up [157]. Another RCT showed that early response is a predictor of sustained remission from binge eating in CBTgsh [158]. A third RCT tested antiobesity medication and shCBT, alone and in combination, and showed that rapid response represents a strong prognostic indicator of clinically meaningful outcomes, even in low-intensity medication and self-help interventions [159].

Some studies show that physical activity counseling and nutritional education added to CBT improve results [160, 161]. However, weight management in comorbid obesity and BED remains a challenge and the best approach has yet to be found [144].

Pharmacotherapy for ED has been the subject of many literature reviews [121, 137, 138, 162–170]. Adverse effects limit clinical utility of some drugs (e.g., tricyclic antidepressants and topiramate), attrition and placebo-responder rates are usually high, binge eating enduring abstinence rates are relatively low, weight loss is mostly unimportant, and long-term effects are largely unknown. Nevertheless, pharmacological therapy may play an ancillary role in the treatment of ED associated with obesity. In particular, it may be an adjunctive treatment for patients who have unsatisfactory response to psychosocial interventions alone and/or suffer from comorbid psychiatric disorders [13, 168, 170].

To go into more detail, many agents can improve BN symptoms. Selective serotonin reuptake inhibitors (SSRIs) are the most prescribed class of drugs [121], but at present fluoxetine (60 mg/die) is the only medicine approved for this indication by the Food and Drug Administration (FDA) and European Medicines Agency (EMA).

As regards BED, several drugs have shown evidence of some therapeutic value, and in some cases pharmacotherapy may be a useful component of a multidimensional treatment approach (see Table 8.3). The medication dosage is usually at the high end of the recommended range. Fluoxetine was tested in several trials for BED with positive results on binge eating frequency, but weight loss was modest [102, 171–176]. Topiramate – an anticonvulsant drug that causes decreased appetite and weight – was titrated from 25 mg/day to a maximum of 600 mg/day in several RCTs for BED and was associated with a significant reduction in binge frequency and a small but significant reduction in BMI; however, adverse effects (e.g., paresthesias, cognitive impairment, somnolence, headache, nausea, and gastrointestinal distress) were frequent and discontinuation rates were high [110–112, 177, 178].

Some studies have examined the added benefit of drugs and other interventions. Adding fluoxetine to psychological interventions produced inconsistent results on BED symptoms and BMI [173, 176, 179–181]. Conversely, topiramate improved the efficacy of CBT increasing binge remission and weight loss [112] and the addition of orlistat to behavioral treatments for patients with BED-obesity was associated with greater weight loss than the addition of placebo [109, 182–184].

Amphetamine inhibits the reuptake and enhances the release of dopamine and norepinephrine. Lisdexamfetamine dimesylate is a dextroamphetamine prodrug marketed for the treatment of attention-deficit/hyperactivity disorder (ADHD) in children and adults. Titrated to 50–70 mg/day in patients with BED-obesity lisdexamfetamine was associated with a significant reduction in binge frequency and a modest but significant weight loss. The most commonly encountered adverse events were dry mouth, decreased appetite, insomnia, and headache. Long-term efficacy is still unknown [120, 185]. At present, lisdexamfetamine is the only medicine approved by FDA (but not yet by EMA) for BED.

With regard to NES, there is very limited evidence to suggest that some drugs (e.g., SSRI, melatonergic medications, topiramate), light therapy, and psychological interventions may be useful [186–189].

Among biological therapies, *deep brain stimulation* (DBS) [190, 191], *repetitive transcranial magnetic stimulation* (rTMS) [192], and *prefrontal cortex transcranial direct current stimulation* (tDCS) [193] are recently being studied in ED. Research in this field is still in its early stages.

On a final note, it could be useful to remind that the prevalence of obesity and disordered eating behaviors (e.g., hyperphagia, binge eating, grazing, emotional eating, night eating) is very high in people diagnosed as having a mental illness [86, 194, 195]. Furthermore, most psychotropic drugs (not only antipsychotics but also antidepressants, and mood stabilizers as well) are associated with the potential risk to induce weight gain and obesity-related disorders [196]. A multisite, parallel two-arm RCT showed that a lifestyle intervention can reduce both weight and fasting glucose levels in individuals with serious psychiatric disorders [197].

References

1. American Psychiatric Association (2013) Diagnostic and statistical manual of mental disorders, DSM-5, 5th edn. American Psychiatric Publishing, Arlington
2. Allison KC, Lundgren JD, O'Reardon JP, Geliebter A, Gluck ME, Vinai P, Mitchell JE, Schenck CH, Howell MJ, Crow SJ, Engel S, Latzer Y, Tzischinsky O, Mahowald MW,

Stunkard AJ (2010) Proposed diagnostic criteria for night eating syndrome. Int J Eat Disord 43(3):241–247. doi:10.1002/eat.20693

3. World Health Organization (2010) International statistical classification of diseases and related health problems, 10th revision. Version 2010. World Health Organization. http://apps.who.int/classifications/icd10/browse/2010/en. Accessed 7 Jan 2014

4. Neumark-Sztainer D (2009) The interface between the eating disorders and obesity fields: moving toward a model of shared knowledge and collaboration. Eat Weight Disord 14(1):51–58

5. Day J, Ternouth A, Collier DA (2009) Eating disorders and obesity: two sides of the same coin? Epidemiol Psichiatr Soc 18(2):96–100

6. Krug I, Villarejo C, Jimenez-Murcia S, Perpina C, Vilarrasa N, Granero R, Cebolla A, Botella C, Montserrat-Gil de Bernabe M, Penelo E, Casella S, Islam MA, Orekhova E, Casanueva FF, Karwautz A, Menchon JM, Treasure J, Fernandez-Aranda F (2013) Eating-related environmental factors in underweight eating disorders and obesity: are there common vulnerabilities during childhood and early adolescence? Eur Eat Disord Rev 21(3):202–208. doi:10.1002/erv.2204

7. Cuzzolaro M (2014) Eating and weight disorders: studies on anorexia, bulimia, and obesity turns 19. Eat Weight Disord 19(1):1–2. doi:10.1007/s40519-014-0104-9

8. Ferrari M (2015) Understanding the feasibility of integrating the eating disorders and obesity fields: the beyond obesity and disordered eating in youth (BODY) study. Eat Weight Disord 20(2):257–269. doi:10.1007/s40519-014-0172-x

9. Hebebrand J, Fichter M, Gerber G, Gorg T, Hermann H, Geller F, Schafer H, Remschmidt H, Hinney A (2002) Genetic predisposition to obesity in bulimia nervosa: a mutation screen of the melanocortin-4 receptor gene. Mol Psychiatry 7(6):647–651. doi:10.1038/sj.mp.4001053

10. Fairburn CG, Welch SL, Doll HA, Davies BA, O'Connor ME (1997) Risk factors for bulimia nervosa: a community-based case–control study. Arch Gen Psychiatry 54(6):509–517. doi:10.1001/archpsyc.1997.01830180015003

11. Hudson J, Pope H, Wutman J (1988) Bulimia in obese individuals. J Nerv Ment Dis 176:144–152

12. Mitchell JE, Pyle RL, Eckert ED, Hatsukami D, Soll E (1990) Bulimia nervosa in overweight individuals. J Nerv Ment Dis 178:324–327

13. Hay P, Chinn D, Forbes D, Madden S, Newton R, Sugenor L, Touyz S, Ward W (2014) Royal Australian and New Zealand College of Psychiatrists clinical practice guidelines for the treatment of eating disorders. Aust NZ J Psychiatry 48(11):977–1008. doi:10.1177/0004867414555814

14. Rotella F, Castellini G, Montanelli L, Rotella CM, Faravelli C, Ricca V (2013) Comparison between normal-weight and overweight bulimic patients. Eat Weight Disord 18(4):389–393. doi:10.1007/s40519-013-0053-8

15. Bulik CM, Marcus MD, Zerwas S, Levine MD, La Via M (2012) The changing "weightscape" of bulimia nervosa. Am J Psychiatry 169(10):1031–1036. doi:10.1176/appi.ajp.2012.12010147

16. Lebow J, Sim LA, Kransdorf LN (2015) Prevalence of a history of overweight and obesity in adolescents with restrictive eating disorders. J Adolesc Health 56(1):19–24. doi:10.1016/j.jadohealth.2014.06.005

17. Witt AA, Berkowitz SA, Gillberg C, Lowe MR, Rastam M, Wentz E (2014) Weight suppression and body mass index interact to predict long-term weight outcomes in adolescent-onset anorexia nervosa. J Consult Clin Psychol 82(6):1207–1211. doi:10.1037/a0037484

18. Berner LA, Shaw JA, Witt AA, Lowe MR (2013) The relation of weight suppression and body mass index to symptomatology and treatment response in anorexia nervosa. J Abnorm Psychol 122(3):694–708. doi:10.1037/a0033930

19. Lowe MR, Berner LA, Swanson SA, Clark VL, Eddy KT, Franko DL, Shaw JA, Ross S, Herzog DB (2011) Weight suppression predicts time to remission from bulimia nervosa. J Consult Clin Psychol 79(6):772–776. doi:10.1037/a0025714

20. Zunker C, Crosby RD, Mitchell JE, Wonderlich SA, Peterson CB, Crow SJ (2011) Weight suppression as a predictor variable in treatment trials of bulimia nervosa and binge eating disorder. Int J Eat Disord 44(8):727–730. doi:10.1002/eat.20839

21. Spear BA (2006) Does dieting increase the risk for obesity and eating disorders? J Am Diet Assoc 106(4):523–525. doi:10.1016/j.jada.2006.01.013

22. Stice E, Durant S, Burger KS, Schoeller DA (2011) Weight suppression and risk of future increases in body mass: effects of suppressed resting metabolic rate and energy expenditure. Am J Clin Nutr 94(1):7–11. doi:10.3945/ajcn.110.010025
23. Segal A, Kinoshita Kussunoki D, Larino MA (2004) Post-surgical refusal to eat: anorexia nervosa, bulimia nervosa or a new eating disorder? a case series. Obes Surg 14(3):353–360
24. Marino JM, Ertelt TW, Lancaster K, Steffen K, Peterson L, de Zwaan M, Mitchell JE (2012) The emergence of eating pathology after bariatric surgery: a rare outcome with important clinical implications. Int J Eat Disord 45(2):179–184. doi:10.1002/eat.20891
25. Konttinen H, Peltonen M, Sjostrom L, Carlsson L, Karlsson J (2015) Psychological aspects of eating behavior as predictors of 10-y weight changes after surgical and conventional treatment of severe obesity: results from the swedish obese subjects intervention study. Am J Clin Nutr 101(1):16–24. doi:10.3945/ajcn.114.095182
26. Fairburn CG, Wilson GT (1993) Binge eating: definition and classification. In: Fairburn CG, Wilson GT (eds) Binge eating. Nature assessment and treatment. The Guilford Press, New York, pp 3–14
27. Colles SL, Dixon JB, O'Brien PE (2008) Loss of control is central to psychological disturbance associated with binge eating disorder. Obesity (Silver Spring) 16(3):608–614
28. Leehr EJ, Krohmer K, Schag K, Dresler T, Zipfel S, Giel KE (2015) Emotion regulation model in binge eating disorder and obesity. A systematic review. Neurosci Biobehav Rev 49:125–134. doi:10.1016/j.neubiorev.2014.12.008
29. Munsch S, Meyer AH, Quartier V, Wilhelm FH (2012) Binge eating in binge eating disorder: a breakdown of emotion regulatory process? Psychiatry Res 195(3):118–124. doi:10.1016/j.psychres.2011.07.016
30. Herman CP, Polivy J (1990) From dietary restraint to binge eating: attaching causes to effects. Appetite 14(2):123–125; discussion 142–123
31. Andres A, Saldana C (2014) Body dissatisfaction and dietary restraint influence binge eating behavior. Nutr Res 34(11):944–950. doi:10.1016/j.nutres.2014.09.003
32. Holmes M, Fuller-Tyszkiewicz M, Skouteris H, Broadbent J (2015) Understanding the link between body image and binge eating: a model comparison approach. Eat Weight Disord 20(1):81–89. doi:10.1007/s40519-014-0141-4
33. Spitzer RL (1991) Nonpurging bulimia nervosa and binge eating disorder. Am J Psychiatry 148(8):1097–1098
34. Cuzzolaro M, Vetrone G (2009) Overview of evidence on the underpinnings of binge eating disorder and obesity. In: Dancyger I, Fornari V (eds) Evidence based treatments for eating disorders: children, adolescents and adults. Nova, New York, pp 53–70
35. Mitchell J, Devlin M, de Zwaan M, Crow S, Peterson C (2008) Binge eating disorder. Clinical foundations and treatment, Guilford, New York
36. Araujo DM, Santos GF, Nardi AE (2010) Binge eating disorder and depression: a systematic review. World J Biol Psychiatry 11(2 Pt 2):199–207. doi:10.3109/15622970802563171
37. Ivezaj V, Kalebjian R, Grilo CM, Barnes RD (2014) Comparing weight gain in the year prior to treatment for overweight and obese patients with and without binge eating disorder in primary care. J Psychosom Res 77(2):151–154. doi:10.1016/j.jpsychores.2014.05.006
38. Grilo CM, White MA, Gueorguieva R, Wilson GT, Masheb RM (2013) Predictive significance of the overvaluation of shape/weight in obese patients with binge eating disorder: findings from a randomized controlled trial with 12-month follow-up. Psychol Med 43(6):1335–1344. doi:10.1017/S0033291712002097
39. Vinai P, Da Ros A, Speciale M, Gentile N, Tagliabue A, Vinai P, Bruno C, Vinai L, Studt S, Cardetti S (2015) Psychopathological characteristics of patients seeking for bariatric surgery, either affected or not by binge eating disorder following the criteria of the DSM IV TR and of the DSM 5. Eat Behav 16:1–4. doi:10.1016/j.eatbeh.2014.10.004
40. Barnes RD, Ivezaj V, Grilo CM (2014) An examination of weight bias among treatment-seeking obese patients with and without binge eating disorder. Gen Hosp Psychiatry 36(2):177–180. doi:10.1016/j.genhosppsych.2013.10.011
41. Grilo CM, White MA, Barnes RD, Masheb RM (2013) Psychiatric disorder co-morbidity and correlates in an ethnically diverse sample of obese patients with binge eating disorder in primary care settings. Compr Psychiatry 54(3):209–216. doi:10.1016/j.comppsych.2012.07.012

42. Becker DF, Grilo CM (2011) Childhood maltreatment in women with binge-eating disorder: associations with psychiatric comorbidity, psychological functioning, and eating pathology. Eat Weight Disord 16(2):e113–e120
43. Marek RJ, Ben-Porath YS, Ashton K, Heinberg LJ (2014) Impact of using DSM-5 criteria for diagnosing binge eating disorder in bariatric surgery candidates: change in prevalence rate, demographic characteristics, and scores on the minnesota multiphasic personality inventory--2 restructured form (MMPI-2-RF). Int J Eat Disord 47(5):553–557. doi:10.1002/eat.22268
44. Becker DF, Grilo CM (2015) Comorbidity of mood and substance use disorders in patients with binge-eating disorder: associations with personality disorder and eating disorder pathology. J Psychosom Res 79(2):159–164. doi:10.1016/j.jpsychores.2015.01.016
45. Jones-Corneille LR, Wadden TA, Sarwer DB, Faulconbridge LF, Fabricatore AN, Stack RM, Cottrell FA, Pulcini ME, Webb VL, Williams NN (2012) Axis I psychopathology in bariatric surgery candidates with and without binge eating disorder: results of structured clinical interviews. Obes Surg 22(3):389–397. doi:10.1007/s11695-010-0322-9
46. Becker DF, Masheb RM, White MA, Grilo CM (2010) Psychiatric, behavioral, and attitudinal correlates of avoidant and obsessive-compulsive personality pathology in patients with binge-eating disorder. Compr Psychiatry 51(5):531–537. doi:10.1016/j.comppsych.2009.11.005
47. Friborg O, Martinussen M, Kaiser S, Overgard KT, Martinsen EW, Schmierer P, Rosenvinge JH (2014) Personality disorders in eating disorder not otherwise specified and binge eating disorder: a meta-analysis of comorbidity studies. J Nerv Ment Dis 202(2):119–125. doi:10.1097/NMD.0000000000000080
48. Sandberg RM, Dahl JK, Vedul-Kjelsas E, Engum B, Kulseng B, Marvik R, Eriksen L (2013) Health-related quality of life in obese presurgery patients with and without binge eating disorder, and subdiagnostic binge eating disorders. J Obes 2013:878310. doi:10.1155/2013/878310
49. Agh T, Kovacs G, Pawaskar M, Supina D, Inotai A, Voko Z (2015) Epidemiology, health-related quality of life and economic burden of binge eating disorder: a systematic literature review. Eat Weight Disord 20(1):1–12. doi:10.1007/s40519-014-0173-9
50. Cuzzolaro M, Bellini M, Donini L, Santomassimo C (2008) Binge eating disorder and body uneasiness. Psych Topics 17(2):287–312
51. Grilo CM, Ivezaj V, White MA (2015) Evaluation of the DSM-5 severity indicator for binge eating disorder in a community sample. Behav Res Ther 66:72–76. doi:10.1016/j.brat.2015.01.004
52. Stunkard A (1959) Eating patterns and obesity. Psychiatr Q 33:284–295
53. Stunkard A, Allison K (2003) Binge eating disorder: disorder or marker? Int J Eat Disord 34(Suppl):S107–S116
54. Amianto F, Ottone L, Abbate Daga G, Fassino S (2015) Binge-eating disorder diagnosis and treatment: a recap in front of DSM-5. BMC Psychiatry 15:70. doi:10.1186/s12888-015-0445-6
55. American Psychiatric Association (1994) Diagnostic and statistical manual of mental disorders, DSM IV, 4th edn. American Psychiatric Association, Washington, DC
56. Hudson JI, Hiripi E, Pope HG Jr, Kessler RC (2007) The prevalence and correlates of eating disorders in the National Comorbidity Survey Replication. Biol Psychiatry 61(3):348–358
57. Stice E, Marti CN, Rohde P (2013) Prevalence, incidence, impairment, and course of the proposed DSM-5 eating disorder diagnoses in an 8-year prospective community study of young women. J Abnorm Psychol 122(2):445–457. doi:10.1037/a0030679
58. Faravelli C, Ravaldi C, Truglia E, Zucchi T, Cosci F, Ricca V (2006) Clinical epidemiology of eating disorders: results from the Sesto Fiorentino study. Psychother Psychosom 75(6):376–383
59. Dahl JK, Eriksen L, Vedul-Kjelsas E, Strommen M, Kulseng B, Marvik R, Holen A (2010) Prevalence of all relevant eating disorders in patients waiting for bariatric surgery: a comparison between patients with and without eating disorders. Eat Weight Disord 15(4):e247–e255
60. Allison KC, Wadden TA, Sarwer DB, Fabricatore AN, Crerand CE, Gibbons LM, Stack RM, Stunkard AJ, Williams NN (2006) Night eating syndrome and binge eating disorder among persons seeking bariatric surgery: prevalence and related features. Obesity (Silver Spring) 14(Suppl 2):77S–82S

61. Mitchell JE, King WC, Courcoulas A, Dakin G, Elder K, Engel S, Flum D, Kalarchian M, Khandelwal S, Pender J, Pories W, Wolfe B (2015) Eating behavior and eating disorders in adults before bariatric surgery. Int J Eat Disord 48(2):215–222. doi:10.1002/eat.22275

62. Parker K, Brennan L (2015) Measurement of disordered eating in bariatric surgery candidates: a systematic review of the literature. Obes Res Clin Pract 9(1):12–25. doi:10.1016/j.orcp.2014.01.005

63. Heymsfield SB, Avena NM, Baier L, Brantley P, Bray GA, Burnett LC, Butler MG, Driscoll DJ, Egli D, Elmquist J, Forster JL, Goldstone AP, Gourash LM, Greenway FL, Han JC, Kane JG, Leibel RL, Loos RJ, Scheimann AO, Roth CL, Seeley RJ, Sheffield V, Tauber M, Vaisse C, Wang L, Waterland RA, Wevrick R, Yanovski JA, Zinn AR (2014) Hyperphagia: current concepts and future directions proceedings of the 2nd international conference on hyperphagia. Obesity (Silver Spring) 22(Suppl 1):S1–S17. doi:10.1002/oby.20646

64. Kweh FA, Miller JL, Sulsona CR, Wasserfall C, Atkinson M, Shuster JJ, Goldstone AP, Driscoll DJ (2015) Hyperghrelinemia in Prader-Willi syndrome begins in early infancy long before the onset of hyperphagia. Am J Med Genet A 167A(1):69–79. doi:10.1002/ajmg.a.36810

65. Conceição EM, Mitchell JE, Engel SG, Machado PPP, Lancaster K, Wonderlich SA (2014) What is "grazing"? reviewing its definition, frequency, clinical characteristics, and impact on bariatric surgery outcomes, and proposing a standardized definition. Surg Obes Relat Dis 10(5):973–982. doi:10.1016/j.soard.2014.05.002

66. Conceicao EM, Crosby R, Mitchell JE, Engel SG, Wonderlich SA, Simonich HK, Peterson CB, Crow SJ, Le Grange D (2013) Picking or nibbling: frequency and associated clinical features in bulimia nervosa, anorexia nervosa, and binge eating disorder. Int J Eat Disord 46(8):815–818. doi:10.1002/eat.22167

67. Zunker C, Karr T, Saunders R, Mitchell JE (2012) Eating behaviors post-bariatric surgery: a qualitative study of grazing. Obes Surg 22(8):1225–1231. doi:10.1007/s11695-012-0647-7

68. Kofman MD, Lent MR, Swencionis C (2010) Maladaptive eating patterns, quality of life, and weight outcomes following gastric bypass: results of an internet survey. Obesity (Silver Spring) 18(10):1938–1943. doi:10.1038/oby.2010.27

69. Saunders R (2004) "Grazing": a high-risk behavior. Obes Surg 14(1):98–102. doi:10.1381/096089204772787374

70. Colles SL, Dixon JB, O'Brien PE (2008) Grazing and loss of control related to eating: two high-risk factors following bariatric surgery. Obesity (Silver Spring) 16(3):615–622. doi:10.1038/oby.2007.101

71. Levin ME, Dalrymple K, Himes S, Zimmerman M (2014) Which facets of mindfulness are related to problematic eating among patients seeking bariatric surgery? Eat Behav 15(2):298–305. doi:10.1016/j.eatbeh.2014.03.012

72. Duarte C, Pinto-Gouveia J (2015) Returning to emotional eating: the emotional eating scale psychometric properties and associations with body image flexibility and binge eating. Eat Weight Disord. doi:10.1007/s40519-015-0186-z

73. van Strien T, Cebolla A, Etchemendy E, Gutierrez-Maldonado J, Ferrer-Garcia M, Botella C, Banos R (2013) Emotional eating and food intake after sadness and joy. Appetite 66:20–25. doi:10.1016/j.appet.2013.02.016

74. Raspopow K, Abizaid A, Matheson K, Anisman H (2014) Anticipation of a psychosocial stressor differentially influences ghrelin, cortisol and food intake among emotional and non-emotional eaters. Appetite 74:35–43. doi:10.1016/j.appet.2013.11.018

75. Labarthe A, Fiquet O, Hassouna R, Zizzari P, Lanfumey L, Ramoz N, Grouselle D, Epelbaum J, Tolle V (2014) Ghrelin-derived peptides: a link between appetite/reward, GH axis, and psychiatric disorders? Front Endocrinol 5:163. doi:10.3389/fendo.2014.00163

76. Weingarten HP, Elston D (1990) The phenomenology of food cravings. Appetite 15(3): 231–246

77. Weingarten HP, Elston D (1991) Food cravings in a college population. Appetite 17(3). 167–175

78. Potenza MN, Grilo CM (2014) How relevant is food craving to obesity and its treatment? Front Psychiatry 5:164. doi:10.3389/fpsyt.2014.00164

79. Werthmann J, Jansen A, Roefs A (2015) Worry or craving? a selective review of evidence for food-related attention biases in obese individuals, eating-disorder patients, restrained eaters and healthy samples. Proc Nutr Soc 74(2):99–114. doi:10.1017/S0029665114001451

80. Ziauddeen H, Fletcher PC (2013) Is food addiction a valid and useful concept? Obes Rev 14(1):19–28. doi:10.1111/j.1467-789X.2012.01046.x

81. Smith DG, Robbins TW (2013) The neurobiological underpinnings of obesity and binge eating: a rationale for adopting the food addiction model. Biol Psychiatry 73(9):804–810. doi:10.1016/j.biopsych.2012.08.026

82. Volkow ND, Wang GJ, Tomasi D, Baler RD (2013) Obesity and addiction: neurobiological overlaps. Obes Rev 14(1):2–18. doi:10.1111/j.1467-789X.2012.01031.x

83. Schulte EM, Joyner MA, Potenza MN, Grilo CM, Gearhardt AN (2015) Current considerations regarding food addiction. Curr Psychiatry Rep 17(4):563. doi:10.1007/s11920-015-0563-3

84. Balodis IM, Grilo CM, Kober H, Worhunsky PD, White MA, Stevens MC, Pearlson GD, Potenza MN (2014) A pilot study linking reduced fronto-striatal recruitment during reward processing to persistent bingeing following treatment for binge-eating disorder. Int J Eat Disord 47(4):376–384. doi:10.1002/eat.22204

85. Gearhardt AN, White MA, Masheb RM, Grilo CM (2013) An examination of food addiction in a racially diverse sample of obese patients with binge eating disorder in primary care settings. Compr Psychiatry 54(5):500–505. doi:10.1016/j.comppsych.2012.12.009

86. Cuzzolaro M (2013) Psychiatric aspects. In: Capodaglio P, Faintuch J, Liuzzi A (eds) Disabling obesity. From determinants to health care models. Springer, Heidelberg, pp 183–197. doi:10.1007/978-3-642-35972-9_10

87. Gearhardt AN, Corbin WR, Brownell KD (2009) Preliminary validation of the yale food addiction scale. Appetite 52(2):430–436. doi:10.1016/j.appet.2008.12.003

88. Gearhardt AN, Yokum S, Orr PT, Stice E, Corbin WR, Brownell KD (2011) Neural correlates of food addiction. Arch Gen Psychiatry 68(8):808–816. doi:10.1001/archgenpsychiatry.2011.32

89. Royal S, Wnuk S, Warwick K, Hawa R, Sockalingam S (2015) Night eating and loss of control over eating in bariatric surgery candidates. J Clin Psychol Med Settings 22(1):14–19. doi:10.1007/s10880-014-9411-6

90. Cleator J, Judd P, James M, Abbott J, Sutton CJ, Wilding JP (2014) Characteristics and perspectives of night-eating behaviour in a severely obese population. Clin Obes 4(1):30 38. doi:10.1111/cob.12037

91. Fairburn CG, Cooper Z, O'Connor ME (2008) Eating disorder examination (Edition 16.0D). In: Fairburn CG (ed) Cognitive behavior therapy and eating disorders. The Guilford Press, New York, pp 265–308

92. Gormally J, Black S, Daston S, Rardin D (1982) The assessment of binge eating severity among obese persons. Addict Behav 7:47–55

93. Cuzzolaro M, Vetrone G, Marano G, Garfinkel PE (2006) The Body Uneasiness Test (BUT): development and validation of a new body image assessment scale. Eat Weight Disord 11(1):1–13

94. Marano G, Cuzzolaro M, Vetrone G, Garfinkel PE, Temperilli F, Spera G, Dalle Grave R, Calugi S, Marchesini G (2007) Validating the Body Uneasiness Test (BUT) in obese patients. Eat Weight Disord 12(2):70–82

95. Yanovski SZ, Marcus MD, Wadden TA, Walsh BT (2014) The questionnaire on eating and weight patterns-5: an updated screening instrument for binge eating disorder. Int J Eat Disord 48(3):259–261. doi:10.1002/eat.22372

96. Hill LS, Reid F, Morgan JF, Lacey JH (2010) SCOFF, the development of an eating disorder screening questionnaire. Int J Eat Disord 43(4):344–351. doi:10.1002/eat.20679

97. Innamorati M, Imperatori C, Manzoni GM, Lamis DA, Castelnuovo G, Tamburello A, Tamburello S, Fabbricatore M (2015) Psychometric properties of the Italian yale food addiction scale in overweight and obese patients. Eat Weight Disord 20(1):119–127. doi:10.1007/s40519-014-0142-3

98. Laederach-Hofmann K, Graf C, Horber F, Lippuner K, Lederer S, Michel R, Schneider M (1999) Imipramine and diet counseling with psychological support in the treatment of obese

binge eaters: a randomized, placebo-controlled double-blind study. Int J Eat Disord 26(3):231–244

99. McCann UD, Agras WS (1990) Successful treatment of nonpurging bulimia nervosa with desipramine: a double-blind, placebo-controlled study. Am J Psychiatry 147(11):1509–1513

100. McElroy SL, Hudson JI, Malhotra S, Welge JA, Nelson EB, Keck PE Jr (2003) Citalopram in the treatment of binge-eating disorder: a placebo-controlled trial. J Clin Psychiatry 64(7):807–813

101. Guerdjikova AI, McElroy SL, Kotwal R, Welge JA, Nelson E, Lake K, Alessio DD, Keck PE Jr (2008) High-dose escitalopram in the treatment of binge-eating disorder with obesity: a placebo-controlled monotherapy trial. Hum Psychopharmacol 23(1):1–11

102. Arnold LM, McElroy SL, Hudson JI, Welge JA, Bennett AJ, Keck PE (2002) A placebo-controlled, randomized trial of fluoxetine in the treatment of binge-eating disorder. J Clin Psychiatry 63(11):1028–1033

103. Hudson JI, McElroy SL, Raymond NC, Crow S, Keck PE Jr, Carter WP, Mitchell JE, Strakowski SM, Pope HG Jr, Coleman BS, Jonas JM (1998) Fluvoxamine in the treatment of binge-eating disorder: a multicenter placebo-controlled, double-blind trial. Am J Psychiatry 155(12):1756–1762

104. Pearlstein T, Spurrell E, Hohlstein L, Gurney V, Read J, Fuchs C, Keller M (2003) A double-blind placebo-controlled trial of fluvoxamine in binge eating disorder: a high placebo response. Arch Womens Ment Health 6(2):147–151

105. McElroy SL, Casuto LS, Nelson EB, Lake KA, Soutullo CA, Keck PE Jr, Hudson JI (2000) Placebo-controlled trial of sertraline in the treatment of binge eating disorder. Am J Psychiatry 157(6):1004–1006

106. McElroy SL, Guerdjikova A, Kotwal R, Welge JA, Nelson EB, Lake KA, Keck PE Jr, Hudson JI (2007) Atomoxetine in the treatment of binge-eating disorder: a randomized placebo-controlled trial. J Clin Psychiatry 68(3):390–398

107. Malhotra S, King KH, Welge JA, Brusman-Lovins L, McElroy SL (2002) Venlafaxine treatment of binge-eating disorder associated with obesity: a series of 35 patients. J Clin Psychiatry 63(9):802–806

108. Guerdjikova AI, McElroy SL, Winstanley EL, Nelson EB, Mori N, McCoy J, Keck PE Jr, Hudson JI (2012) Duloxetine in the treatment of binge eating disorder with depressive disorders: a placebo-controlled trial. Int J Eat Disord 45(2):281–289. doi:10.1002/eat.20946

109. Golay A, Laurent-Jaccard A, Habicht F, Gachoud JP, Chabloz M, Kammer A, Schutz Y (2005) Effect of orlistat in obese patients with binge eating disorder. Obes Res 13(10): 1701–1708

110. McElroy SL, Arnold LM, Shapira NA, Keck PE Jr, Rosenthal NR, Karim MR, Kamin M, Hudson JI (2003) Topiramate in the treatment of binge eating disorder associated with obesity: a randomized, placebo-controlled trial. Am J Psychiatry 160(2):255–261

111. McElroy SL, Hudson JI, Capece JA, Beyers K, Fisher AC, Rosenthal NR, Topiramate Binge Eating Disorder Research Group (2007) Topiramate for the treatment of binge eating disorder associated with obesity: a placebo-controlled study. Biol Psychiatry 61(9):1039–1048. doi:10.1016/j.biopsych.2006.08.008

112. Claudino AM, de Oliveira IR, Appolinario JC, Cordas TA, Duchesne M, Sichieri R, Bacaltchuk J (2007) Double-blind, randomized, placebo-controlled trial of topiramate plus cognitive-behavior therapy in binge-eating disorder. J Clin Psychiatry 68(9):1324–1332

113. McElroy SL, Shapira NA, Arnold LM, Keck PE, Rosenthal NR, Wu SC, Capece JA, Fazzio L, Hudson JI (2004) Topiramate in the long-term treatment of binge-eating disorder associated with obesity. J Clin Psychiatry 65(11):1463–1469

114. McElroy SL, Kotwal R, Guerdjikova AI, Welge JA, Nelson EB, Lake KA, D'Alessio DA, Keck PE, Hudson JI (2006) Zonisamide in the treatment of binge eating disorder with obesity: a randomized controlled trial. J Clin Psychiatry 67(12):1897–1906

115. Ricca V, Castellini G, Lo Sauro C, Rotella CM, Faravelli C (2009) Zonisamide combined with cognitive behavioral therapy in binge eating disorder: a One-year follow-up study. Psychiatry (Edgmont) 6(11):23–28

116. Guerdjikova AI, McElroy SL, Welge JA, Nelson E, Keck PE, Hudson JI (2009) Lamotrigine in the treatment of binge-eating disorder with obesity: a randomized, placebo-controlled monotherapy trial. Int Clin Psychopharmacol 24(3):150–158. doi:10.1097/YIC.0b013e328329c7b5

117. Corwin RL, Boan J, Peters KF, Ulbrecht JS (2012) Baclofen reduces binge eating in a double-blind, placebo-controlled, crossover study. Behav Pharmacol 23(5–6):616–625. doi:10.1097/FBP.0b013e328357bd62

118. McElroy SL, Guerdjikova AI, Winstanley EL, O'Melia AM, Mori N, Keck PE Jr, Hudson JI (2011) Sodium oxybate in the treatment of binge eating disorder: an open-label, prospective study. Int J Eat Disord 44(3):262–268. doi:10.1002/eat.20798

119. McElroy SL, Guerdjikova AI, Winstanley EL, O'Melia AM, Mori N, McCoy J, Keck PE Jr, Hudson JI (2011) Acamprosate in the treatment of binge eating disorder: a placebo-controlled trial. Int J Eat Disord 44(1):81–90. doi:10.1002/eat.20876

120. McElroy SL, Hudson JI, Mitchell JE, Wilfley D, Ferreira-Cornwell MC, Gao J, Wang J, Whitaker T, Jonas J, Gasior M (2015) Efficacy and safety of lisdexamfetamine for treatment of adults with moderate to severe binge-eating disorder: a randomized clinical trial. JAMA Psychiatry 72(3):235–246. doi:10.1001/jamapsychiatry.2014.2162

121. Mitchell JE, Roerig J, Steffen K (2013) Biological therapies for eating disorders. Int J Eat Disord 46(5):470–477. doi:10.1002/eat.22104

122. Mitchell J, de Zwaan M (eds) (2005) Bariatric surgery. A guide for mental health professionals. Routledge, New York

123. Basdevant A, Guy-Grand B (eds) (2004) Médecine de l'obésité. Flammarion, Paris

124. Wadden T, Stunkard A (eds) (2002) Handbook of obesity treatment. Guilford, New York

125. Ashton K, Drerup M, Windover A, Heinberg L (2009) Brief, four-session group CBT reduces binge eating behaviors among bariatric surgery candidates. Surg Obes Relat Dis 5(2):257–262. doi:10.1016/j.soard.2009.01.005

126. Saunders R (1999) Binge eating in gastric bypass patients before surgery. Obes Surg 9(1):72–76. doi:10.1381/096089299765553845

127. Gade H, Friborg O, Rosenvinge JH, Smastuen MC, Hjelmesaeth J (2015) The impact of a preoperative Cognitive Behavioural Therapy (CBT) on dysfunctional eating behaviours, affective symptoms and body weight 1 year after bariatric surgery: a randomised controlled trial. Obes Surg. doi:10.1007/s11695-015-1673-z

128. Saunders R (2004) Post-surgery group therapy for gastric bypass patients. Obes Surg 14(8):1128–1131. doi:10.1381/0960892041975532

129. Meany G, Conceicao E, Mitchell JE (2014) Binge eating, binge eating disorder and loss of control eating: effects on weight outcomes after bariatric surgery. Eur Eat Disord Rev 22(2):87–91. doi:10.1002/erv.2273

130. Raevuori A, Suokas J, Haukka J, Gissler M, Linna M, Grainger M, Suvisaari J (2014) Highly increased risk of type 2 diabetes in patients with binge eating disorder and bulimia nervosa. Int J Eat Disord. doi:10.1002/eat.22334

131. Donini LM, Cuzzolaro M, Spera G, Badiali M, Basso N, Bollea MR, Bosello O, Brunani A, Busetto L, Cairella G, Cannella C, Capodaglio P, Carbonelli MG, Castellaneta E, Castra R, Clini E, Contaldo F, Dalla Ragione L, Dalle Grave R, D'Andrea F, Del Balzo V, De Cristofaro P, Di Flaviano E, Fassino S, Ferro AM, Forestieri P, Franzoni E, Gentile MG, Giustini A, Jacoangeli F, Lubrano C, Lucchin L, Manara F, Marangi G, Marcelli M, Marchesini G, Marri G, Marrocco W, Melchionda N, Mezzani B, Migliaccio P, Muratori F, Nizzoli U, Ostuzzi R, Panzolato G, Pasanisi F, Persichetti P, Petroni ML, Pontieri V, Prosperi E, Renna C, Rovera G, Santini F, Saraceni V, Savina C, Scuderi N, Silecchia G, Strollo F, Todisco P, Tubili C, Ugolini G, Zamboni M (2010) Obesity and eating disorders. Indications for the different levels of care. An Italian expert consensus document. Eat Weight Disord 15(1–2 Suppl):1–31

132. National Institute for Health and Care Excellence (2004) Eating disorders: Core interventions in the treatment and management of anorexia nervosa, bulimia nervosa and related eating disorders. NICE Clinical Guideline 9, http://www.nice.org.uk/guidance/cg9

133. American Psychiatric Association (2006) Practice guideline for the treatment of patients with eating disorders (third edition). Am J Psychiatry 163(July Suppl):1–54

134. National Institute for Health and Care Excellence (2014) Obesity: identification, assessment and management of overweight and obesity in children, young people and adults. NICE Clinical Guideline 189, http://www.nice.org.uk/guidance/cg189

135. Apovian C, Aronne L, Bessesen D, McDonnell M, Murad M, Pagotto U, Ryan D, Still C (2015) Pharmacological management of obesity: an endocrine society clinical practice guideline. J Clin Endocrinol Metab 100(2):342–362. doi:10.1210/jc.2014-3415

136. National Health and Medical Research Council (2013) Clinical practice guidelines for the management of overweight and obesity in adults, adolescents and children in Australia. National Health and Medical Research Council. http://www.nhmrc.gov.au/guidelines/publications/n57, Melbourne

137. Vocks S, Tuschen-Caffier B, Pietrowsky R, Rustenbach SJ, Kersting A, Herpertz S (2010) Meta-analysis of the effectiveness of psychological and pharmacological treatments for binge eating disorder. Int J Eat Disord 43(3):205–217. doi:10.1002/eat.20696

138. Wilson GT (2011) Treatment of binge eating disorder. Psychiatr Clin North Am 34(4):773–783. doi:10.1016/j.psc.2011.08.011

139. O'Reilly GA, Cook L, Spruijt-Metz D, Black DS (2014) Mindfulness-based interventions for obesity-related eating behaviours: a literature review. Obes Rev 15(6):453–461. doi:10.1111/obr.12156

140. Beintner I, Jacobi C, Schmidt UH (2014) Participation and outcome in manualized self-help for bulimia nervosa and binge eating disorder – a systematic review and metaregression analysis. Clin Psychol Rev 34(2):158–176. doi:10.1016/j.cpr.2014.01.003

141. Lock J (2015) An update on evidence-based psychosocial treatments for eating disorders in children and adolescents. J Clin Child Adolesc Psychol 44(5):707–721. doi:10.1080/15374416.2014.971458

142. Spielmans GI, Benish SG, Marin C, Bowman WM, Menster M, Wheeler AJ (2013) Specificity of psychological treatments for bulimia nervosa and binge eating disorder? a meta-analysis of direct comparisons. Clin Psychol Rev 33(3):460–469. doi:10.1016/j.cpr.2013.01.008

143. Ramacciotti CE, Coli E, Marazziti D, Segura-Garcia C, Brambilla F, Piccinni A, Dell'osso L (2013) Therapeutic options for binge eating disorder. Eat Weight Disord 18(1):3–9. doi:10.1007/s40519-013-0003-5

144. Hay P (2013) A systematic review of evidence for psychological treatments in eating disorders: 2005–2012. Int J Eat Disord 46(5):462–469. doi:10.1002/eat.22103

145. Crow SJ (2003) Group interpersonal psychotherapy may be as effective as group cognitive behavioural therapy for overweight people with binge eating disorder. Evid Based Ment Health 6(2):56

146. Wilfley DE, Welch RR, Stein RI, Spurrell EB, Cohen LR, Saelens BE, Dounchis JZ, Frank MA, Wiseman CV, Matt GE (2002) A randomized comparison of group cognitive-behavioral therapy and group interpersonal psychotherapy for the treatment of overweight individuals with binge-eating disorder. Arch Gen Psychiatry 59(8):713–721

147. Agras WS, Telch CF, Arnow B, Eldredge K, Detzer MJ, Henderson J, Marnell M (1995) Does interpersonal therapy help patients with binge eating disorder who fail to respond to cognitive-behavioral therapy? J Consult Clin Psychol 63(3):356–360

148. Wilson GT, Wilfley DE, Agras WS, Bryson SW (2010) Psychological treatments of binge eating disorder. Arch Gen Psychiatry 67(1):94–101. doi:10.1001/archgenpsychiatry.2009.170

149. Ricca V, Castellini G, Mannucci E, Lo Sauro C, Ravaldi C, Rotella CM, Faravelli C (2010) Comparison of individual and group cognitive behavioral therapy for binge eating disorder. A randomized, three-year follow-up study. Appetite 55(3):656–665. doi:10.1016/j.appet.2010.09.019, S0195-6663(10)00517-9 [pii]

150. Brauhardt A, de Zwaan M, Herpertz S, Zipfel S, Svaldi J, Friederich HC, Hilbert A (2014) Therapist adherence in individual cognitive-behavioral therapy for binge-eating disorder: assessment, course, and predictors. Behav Res Ther 61:55–60. doi:10.1016/j.brat.2014.07.014

151. Fischer S, Meyer AH, Dremmel D, Schlup B, Munsch S (2014) Short-term cognitive-behavioral therapy for binge eating disorder: long-term efficacy and predictors of long-term treatment success. Behav Res Ther 58:36–42. doi:10.1016/j.brat.2014.04.007

152. Fairburn CG, Cooper Z, Doll HA, O'Connor ME, Bohn K, Hawker DM, Wales JA, Palmer RL (2009) Transdiagnostic cognitive-behavioral therapy for patients with eating disorders: a two-site trial with 60-week follow-up. Am J Psychiatry 166(3):311–319. doi:10.1176/appi.ajp.2008.08040608
153. Godfrey KM, Gallo LC, Afari N (2015) Mindfulness-based interventions for binge eating: a systematic review and meta-analysis. J Behav Med 38(2):348–362. doi:10.1007/s10865-014-9610-5
154. Telch CF, Agras WS, Linehan MM (2001) Dialectical behavior therapy for binge eating disorder. J Consult Clin Psychol 69(6):1061–1065
155. Safer DL, Robinson AH, Jo B (2010) Outcome from a randomized controlled trial of group therapy for binge eating disorder: comparing dialectical behavior therapy adapted for binge eating to an active comparison group therapy. Behav Ther 41(1):106–120. doi:10.1016/j.beth.2009.01.006
156. Masson PC, von Ranson KM, Wallace LM, Safer DL (2013) A randomized wait-list controlled pilot study of dialectical behaviour therapy guided self-help for binge eating disorder. Behav Res Ther 51(11):723–728. doi:10.1016/j.brat.2013.08.001
157. Safer DL, Joyce EE (2011) Does rapid response to two group psychotherapies for binge eating disorder predict abstinence? Behav Res Ther 49(5):339–345. doi:10.1016/j.brat.2011.03.001
158. Hilbert A, Hildebrandt T, Agras WS, Wilfley DE, Wilson GT (2015) Rapid response in psychological treatments for binge eating disorder. J Consult Clin Psychol 83(3):649–654. doi:10.1037/ccp0000018
159. Grilo CM, White MA, Masheb RM, Gueorguieva R (2015) Predicting meaningful outcomes to medication and self-help treatments for binge-eating disorder in primary care: the significance of early rapid response. J Consult Clin Psychol 83(2):387–394. doi:10.1037/a0038635
160. Vancampfort D, Probst M, Adriaens A, Pieters G, De Hert M, Stubbs B, Soundy A, Vanderlinden J (2014) Changes in physical activity, physical fitness, self-perception and quality of life following a 6-month physical activity counseling and cognitive behavioral therapy program in outpatients with binge eating disorder. Psychiatry Res 219(2):361–366. doi:10.1016/j.psychres.2014.05.016
161. Fossati M, Amati F, Painot D, Reiner M, Haenni C, Golay A (2004) Cognitive-behavioral therapy with simultaneous nutritional and physical activity education in obese patients with binge eating disorder. Eat Weight Disord 9(2):134–138
162. Goracci A, di Volo S, Casamassima F, Bolognesi S, Benbow J, Fagiolini A (2015) Pharmacotherapy of binge-eating disorder: a review. J Addict Med 9(1):1–19. doi:10.1097/ADM.0000000000000089
163. Brownley KA, Peat CM, La Via M, Bulik CM (2015) Pharmacological approaches to the management of binge eating disorder. Drugs 75(1):9–32. doi:10.1007/s40265-014-0327-0
164. Reas DL, Grilo CM (2014) Current and emerging drug treatments for binge eating disorder. Expert Opin Emerg Drugs 19(1):99–142. doi:10.1517/14728214.2014.879291
165. Stefano SC, Bacaltchuk J, Blay SL, Appolinario JC (2008) Antidepressants in short-term treatment of binge eating disorder: systematic review and meta-analysis. Eat Behav 9(2):129–136
166. Hay PJ, Claudino AM (2012) Clinical psychopharmacology of eating disorders: a research update. Int J Neuropsychopharmacol 15(2):209–222. doi:10.1017/S1461145711000460
167. McElroy SL, Guerdjikova AI, Mori N, Keck PE Jr (2015) Psychopharmacologic treatment of eating disorders: emerging findings. Curr Psychiatry Rep 17(5):35. doi:10.1007/s11920-015-0573-1
168. Flament MF, Bissada H, Spettigue W (2012) Evidence-based pharmacotherapy of eating disorders. Int J Neuropsychopharmacol 15(2):189–207. doi:10.1017/S1461145711000381
169. Blom TJ, Mingione CJ, Guerdjikova AI, Keck PE Jr, Welge JA, McElroy SL (2014) Placebo response in binge eating disorder: a pooled analysis of 10 clinical trials from one research group. Eur Eat Disord Rev 22(2):140–146. doi:10.1002/erv.2277
170. Aigner M, Treasure J, Kaye W, Kasper S (2011) World Federation of Societies of Biological Psychiatry (WFSBP) guidelines for the pharmacological treatment of eating disorders. World J Biol Psychia 12(6):400–443. doi:10.3109/15622975.2011.602720
171. Greeno CG, Wing RR (1996) A double blind, placebo-controlled trial of the effect of fluoxetine on dietary intake in overweight women with and without binge-eating disorder. Am J Clin Nutr 64(3):267–273

172. Devlin MJ, Goldfein JA, Petkova E, Jiang H, Raizman PS, Wolk S, Mayer L, Carino J, Bellace D, Kamenetz C, Dobrow I, Walsh BT (2005) Cognitive behavioral therapy and fluoxetine as adjuncts to group behavioral therapy for binge eating disorder. Obes Res 13(6):1077–1088

173. Grilo CM, Masheb RM, Wilson GT (2005) Efficacy of cognitive behavioral therapy and fluoxetine for the treatment of binge eating disorder: a randomized double-blind placebo-controlled comparison. Biol Psychiatry 57(3):301–309

174. Devlin MJ, Goldfein JA, Petkova E, Liu L, Walsh BT (2007) Cognitive behavioral therapy and fluoxetine for binge eating disorder: two-year follow-up. Obesity (Silver Spring) 15(7):1702–1709. doi:10.1038/oby.2007.203

175. Leombruni P, Piero A, Lavagnino L, Brustolin A, Campisi S, Fassino S (2008) A randomized, double-blind trial comparing sertraline and fluoxetine 6-month treatment in obese patients with binge eating disorder. Prog Neuropsychopharmacol Biol Psychiatry 32(6):1599–1605. doi:10.1016/j.pnpbp.2008.06.005

176. Grilo CM, Crosby RD, Wilson GT, Masheb RM (2012) 12-month follow-up of fluoxetine and cognitive behavioral therapy for binge eating disorder. J Consult Clin Psychol 80(6):1108–1113. doi:10.1037/a0030061

177. Tata AL, Kockler DR (2006) Topiramate for binge-eating disorder associated with obesity. Ann Pharmacother 40(11):1993–1997. doi:10.1345/aph.1H178

178. Arbaizar B, Gomez-Acebo I, Llorca J (2008) Efficacy of topiramate in bulimia nervosa and binge-eating disorder: a systematic review. Gen Hosp Psychiatry 30(5):471–475. doi:10.1016/j.genhosppsych.2008.02.002

179. Ricca V, Mannucci E, Mezzani B, Moretti S, Di Bernardo M, Bertelli M, Rotella CM, Faravelli C (2001) Fluoxetine and fluvoxamine combined with individual cognitive-behaviour therapy in binge eating disorder: a one-year follow-up study. Psychother Psychosom 70(6):298–306, doi:56270

180. Marcus MD, Wing RR, Ewing L, Kern E, McDermott M, Gooding W (1990) A double-blind, placebo-controlled trial of fluoxetine plus behavior modification in the treatment of obese binge-eaters and non-binge-eaters. Am J Psychiatry 147(7):876–881

181. Molinari E, Baruffi M, Croci M, Marchi S, Petroni ML (2005) Binge eating disorder in obesity: comparison of different therapeutic strategies. Eat Weight Disord 10(3):154–161

182. Grilo CM, Masheb RM, Salant SL (2005) Cognitive behavioral therapy guided self-help and orlistat for the treatment of binge eating disorder: a randomized, double-blind, placebo-controlled trial. Biol Psychiatry 57(10):1193–1201. doi:10.1016/j.biopsych.2005.03.001

183. Grilo CM, Masheb RM (2007) Rapid response predicts binge eating and weight loss in binge eating disorder: findings from a controlled trial of orlistat with guided self-help cognitive behavioral therapy. Behav Res Ther 45(11):2537–2550. doi:10.1016/j.brat.2007.05.010

184. Grilo CM, White MA (2013) Orlistat with behavioral weight loss for obesity with versus without binge eating disorder: randomized placebo-controlled trial at a community mental health center serving educationally and economically disadvantaged Latino/as. Behav Res Ther 51(3):167–175. doi:10.1016/j.brat.2013.01.002

185. Citrome L (2015) Lisdexamfetamine for binge eating disorder in adults: a systematic review of the efficacy and safety profile for this newly approved indication - what is the number needed to treat, number needed to harm and likelihood to be helped or harmed? Int J Clin Pract 69(4):410–421. doi:10.1111/ijcp.12639

186. Kucukgoncu S, Midura M, Tek C (2015) Optimal management of night eating syndrome: challenges and solutions. Neuropsychiatr Dis Treat 11:751–760. doi:10.2147/NDT.S70312

187. Vander Wal JS, Maraldo TM, Vercellone AC, Gagne DA (2015) Education, progressive muscle relaxation therapy, and exercise for the treatment of night eating syndrome. A pilot study. Appetite 89:136–144. doi:10.1016/j.appet.2015.01.024

188. Stunkard A, Lu XY (2010) Rapid changes in night eating: considering mechanisms. Eat Weight Disord 15(1–2):e2–e8

189. Milano W, De Rosa M, Milano L, Capasso A (2012) Night eating syndrome: an overview. J Pharm Pharmacol 64(1):2–10. doi:10.1111/j.2042-7158.2011.01353.x

190. Martire SI, Tran DM, Reichelt AC (2013) Preventing binge eating with deep brain stimulation – can compulsive eating be switched Off? Front Psychiatry 4:168. doi:10.3389/fpsyt.2013.00168

191. Halpern CH, Tekriwal A, Santollo J, Keating JG, Wolf JA, Daniels D, Bale TL (2013) Amelioration of binge eating by nucleus accumbens shell deep brain stimulation in mice involves D2 receptor modulation. J Neurosci 33(17):7122–7129. doi:10.1523/JNEUROSCI.3237-12.2013

192. Baczynski TP, de Aquino Chaim CH, Nazar BP, Carta MG, Arias-Carrion O, Silva AC, Machado S, Nardi AE (2014) High-frequency rTMS to treat refractory binge eating disorder and comorbid depression: a case report. CNS Neurol Disord Drug Targets 13(5):771–775

193. Kekic M, McClelland J, Campbell I, Nestler S, Rubia K, David AS, Schmidt U (2014) The effects of prefrontal cortex transcranial direct current stimulation (tDCS) on food craving and temporal discounting in women with frequent food cravings. Appetite 78:55–62. doi:10.1016/j.appet.2014.03.010

194. Pagoto S, Bodenlos JS, Kantor L, Gitkind M, Curtin C, Ma Y (2007) Association of major depression and binge eating disorder with weight loss in a clinical setting. Obesity (Silver Spring) 15(11):2557–2559

195. Simon GE, Von Korff M, Saunders K, Miglioretti DL, Crane PK, van Belle G, Kessler RC (2006) Association between obesity and psychiatric disorders in the US adult population. Arch Gen Psychiatry 63(7):824–830. doi:10.1001/archpsyc.63.7.824

196. Domecq JP, Prutsky G, Leppin A, Sonbol MB, Altayar O, Undavalli C, Wang Z, Elraiyah T, Brito JP, Mauck KF, Lababidi MH, Prokop LJ, Asi N, Wei J, Fidahussein S, Montori VM, Murad MH (2015) Clinical review: drugs commonly associated with weight change: a systematic review and meta-analysis. J Clin Endocrinol Metab 100(2):363–370. doi:10.1210/jc.2014-3421

197. Green CA, Yarborough BJ, Leo MC, Yarborough MT, Stumbo SP, Janoff SL, Perrin NA, Nichols GA, Stevens VJ (2014) The STRIDE weight loss and lifestyle intervention for individuals taking antipsychotic medications: a randomized trial. Am J Psychiatry. doi:10.1176/appi.ajp.2014.14020173

Obesity in Pregnancy

9

Annunziata Lapolla and Maria Grazia Dalfrà

9.1 Introduction

Obesity in childbearing age affects an increasing number of women worldwide [1–3], and the increasing prevalence of obesity throughout the world has also been accompanied by an increase in the average weight gained during pregnancy [4].

Since maternal obesity has adverse effects on maternal and fetal outcome, it is important to monitor these pregnancies to prevent or reduce its negative effects and risks.

9.2 Risks Related to Obesity During Pregnancy

9.2.1 Maternal Mortality and Comorbidities

According to Confidential Enquires into Maternal and Child Health (CEMACH) reports, there is a 50 % greater prenatal and peripartum mortality rate in obese mothers with respect to their nonobese counterparts [5]. In addition to maternal death, maternal preconception body mass index (BMI) has been linked to other comorbidities such as gestational diabetes mellitus (GDM) (OR 2.6 and 4.0) [6], gestational hypertension (OR 2.5 and 3.2) [7], preeclampsia (OR 1.6 and 3.3), cesarean section delivery [8], wound breakdowns, and venous thromboembolism.

A study carried out in Northern California reported that women who gained 2.3–10 kg per year in prepregnancy years had a 2.5-fold increased risk of gestational diabetes mellitus (GDM) compared to women whose weight remained stable [6].

A. Lapolla (✉) • M.G. Dalfrà
Department of Medicine – DIMED,
University of Padova, Padova, PD, Italy
e-mail: annunziata.lapolla@unipd.it

© Springer International Publishing Switzerland 2016
P. Sbraccia et al. (eds.), *Clinical Management of Overweight and Obesity:*
Recommendations of the Italian Society of Obesity (SIO),
DOI 10.1007/978-3-319-24532-4_9

Another large study focusing on the risk factors associated to preeclampsia found that the most important ones were: systolic blood pressure at conception, followed by prepregnancy BMI, the number of prior induced or spontaneous abortions, and smoking history (which was protective) [7]. An increase in relative prepregnancy weight (defined as percentage of desired weight for height) was also found to be associated to an increased risk for preeclampsia [7].

9.2.2 Fetal Outcomes

Higher maternal preconception BMI has also been linked to adverse fetal outcomes such as spontaneous abortions, neural tube defects, and macrosomia [8, 9, 19]. Although the overall incidence of spontaneous abortions was low, a meta-analysis found that the risk was greater in obese versus nonobese women (odds ratio [OR] 3.05; 95 % confidence interval [CI], 1.45–6.44) [8]. In a large cohort of infants, maternal obesity was found to be associated to an increased odds ratio of spina bifida (OR 2.09; 95 % CI, 1.63–2.70), heart defects (OR 1.26; 95 % CI, 1.11–1.43), and diaphragmatic hernias (OR 1.41; 95 % CI, 1.01–1.97) [9–18]. Infants born to obese mothers are more likely to be large for gestational age (LGA) or have a birth weight greater than the 90th percentile. When the records of 12,950 deliveries were analyzed, it was found that there was a 17 % prevalence of LGA infants in the obese mothers, a 12 % prevalence in the overweight mothers, and an 11 % prevalence in the nonobese mothers ($P < 0.01$) [10]. Preconception maternal obesity (OR 1.6) and preconception diabetes (OR 4.4) were also found to be independent risk factors for having an LGA infant [10].

9.3 Prepregnancy Care

All women of childbearing age with BMI ≥ 30 (kg/m^2) should be informed about the risks associated with obesity in pregnancy and encouraged to lose weight before becoming pregnant. These efforts should be supported by family planning teams, including primary care general practitioners, gynecologists, and other trained professionals. (*Level of evidence II, Strength of Recommendation B*)

Obese women should be encouraged to lose weight and, if possible, to aim to conceive when their BMI is lower than 30 kg/m^2 [11]. (*Level of Evidence III, Strength of Recommendation B*)

Women with BMI ≥ 30 kg/m^2 who are planning to become pregnant should be advised to take folic acid (5 mg daily) beginning at least one month before conceiving and throughout the first trimester of pregnancy. This supplement has been shown to be effective in reducing the risk of neural tube defects, and this is important given the high incidence of these defects in the offspring of obese women (RR 0.28, 95 % CI 0.13–0.58) [12, 14]. (*Level of Evidence I, Strength of Recommendation A*)

As women with a BMI above 30 kg/m^2 are at higher risk of vitamin D deficiency with respect to their normal-weight counterparts, they should be recommended to take vitamin D (10 micrograms) supplementation throughout pregnancy and lactation [12]. (*Level of evidence II, Strength of Recommendation B*)

9.4   Pregnancy Care

Pregnancies complicated by obesity should be managed by a multidisciplinary team consisting of an endocrinologist, a gynecologist, a specialized nurse, an obstetrician, a dietician, and other trained professionals who will, together, attempt to reduce maternal and fetal complications associated with this condition. (*Level of evidence II, Strength of Recommendation A*)

Weight, BMI, and blood pressure should be strictly monitored throughout the pregnancy of obese women.

As obese women have an increased risk of hypertension, preeclampsia, and eclampsia, health care professionals should carefully and frequently monitor blood pressure; frequent monitoring of proteinuria and of renal and hepatic function, which should be repeated as needed, is also recommended during the second trimester [12]. (*Level of evidence II, Strength of Recommendation A*)

As recommended by national and international guidelines, all pregnant women with a prepregnancy BMI ≥ 30 kg/m^2 need to be screened for gestational diabetes mellitus (GDM) [15–17, 20]. (*Level of evidence II Strength of Recommendation B*)

Given the high risk of fetal complications in this population, fetal growth should be closely monitored [12, 15]. (*Level of evidence II, Strength of Recommendation A*)

All obese pregnant women should be assessed during the first antenatal examination and periodically throughout the pregnancy by the obstetrician and the anesthesiologist to foresee difficulties during delivery linked to venous access, anesthesia (local, general), and the risk of thromboembolic events [12]. (*Level of evidence II, Strength of Recommendation A*)

As demonstrated by a series of cohort studies, maternal obesity is associated with increased risk of thromboembolism both during and after pregnancy. Obese pregnant women who have two additional risk factors for thromboembolism should be considered for low molecular weight heparin prophylaxis, which should be continued for 6 weeks after delivery [21]. (*Level of evidence II, Strength of Recommendation B*)

9.5   Nutritional Therapy

In accordance with the Institute of Medicine (IOM) recommendations [4], individualized nutrition consultation should be offered to all obese pregnant women to promote healthy weight gain and an adequate supply of nutrients to the mother and fetus [22].

It is not advisable for obese pregnant women to lose weight during pregnancy [4]. Obese pregnant women are recommended to eat a variety of foods, including five servings of fruit and vegetables daily and a serving of fatty fish weekly to ensure an appropriate supply of nutrients and fetal well-being, [4, 23, 24]. (*Level of evidence III, Strength of Recommendation B*)

Healthy eating and moderate physical activity (not harmful for the infant) interventions have been shown to be effective in preventing excessive weight gain in obese pregnant women [25]. (*Level of evidence II, Strength of Recommendation B*)

9.6   Partum

The type of delivery of obese pregnant women should be carefully evaluated by a multidisciplinary team. It is also recommended that these women give birth in a medical center containing or linked to a neonatal intensive care unit in the event of any neonatal complications.

Early mobilization of these women after delivery should be encouraged, and antibiotic prophylaxis (in obese women undergoing caesarean section) is also recommended to reduce the risk of thromboembolism and postpartum infections. (*Level of evidence II, Strength of Recommendation A*)

9.7   Postnatal

Randomized controlled trials have shown that a structured educational approach that encourages obese women to breastfeed has a positive effect on lactation, both in terms of onset and duration. (*Level of Evidence I, Strength of Recommendation A*)

Monitoring weight gain and nutrition in the attempt to assist these women to achieve an "acceptable" weight after pregnancy and a structured educational approach encouraging physical activity and promoting healthy food choices have proven to be effective measures to reduce body weight after delivery. (*Level of Evidence I, Strength of Recommendation A*)

As weight loss before another pregnancy is begun is recommended, obese women should be encouraged to consult with a weight-reduction specialist. (*Level of evidence II Strength of Recommendation D*)

A 75-g 2-h OGTT should be performed in all obese women who have been diagnosed with gestational diabetes 6–12 weeks after delivery in view of their risk of developing type 2 diabetes. (*Level of Evidence I, Strength of Recommendation A*)

Observational and cohort studies have consistently demonstrated that obese women with gestational diabetes have a higher risk of developing type 2 diabetes after giving birth than do normal-weight women [12].

Obese women diagnosed with GDM but with a normal glucose tolerance test after delivery need to be regularly monitored to prevent or precociously diagnose type 2 diabetes. (*Level of Evidence I, Strength of Recommendation A*)

9.8 Pregnancy After Bariatric Surgery

Women who have undergone restrictive or malabsorptive bariatric procedures who become pregnant need to be cared for by a multidisciplinary health team consisting of an endocrinologist, a gynecologist, the bariatric surgeon, an anaesthetist, a specialized nurse, an obstetrician, and other trained professionals.

Some studies advise waiting 12–24 months after bariatric surgery when the woman has achieved her weight loss goal before trying to conceive so as not to expose the fetus to an *in utero* environment undergoing rapid maternal weight alterations [12, 26]. (*Level of Evidence III, Strength of Recommendation B*)

Given that nutritional deficiencies (in particular in vitamin B12, folate, iron, vitamin D, and calcium) are common after bariatric surgery, oral supplements are strongly recommended [12, 26]. (*Level of Evidence II, Strength of Recommendation B*)

Partial or complete band deflation may be necessary in pregnant women who have undergone laparoscopic-adjustable gastric banding if they experience nausea and vomiting. Intestinal obstruction, which can occur after gastric bypass surgery, is a complication that requires even greater clinical surveillance during pregnancy [12]. (*Level of Evidence III, Strength of Recommendation B*)

9.9 Education of Health Professionals

All health professionals working in a team that manages obese pregnant women need to be knowledgeable about maternal nutrition and its impact on fetal growth and development; they also need to be aware of the special assistance obese pregnant women require [12]. (*Level of Evidence III, Strength of Recommendation B*)

References

1. Flegal KM, Carroll MD, Ogden CL et al (2010) Prevalence and trends in obesity among US adults, 1999-2008. JAMA 303(3):235–241
2. World Health Organization (2006) Fact sheets no 311. WHO, Geneva
3. World Health Organization (2009) Global data base on body mass index. WHO, Geneva
4. Rasmussen KM, Yaktine AL, Committee to reexamine IOM Pregnancy weight guidelines (2009) Weight gain during pregnancy. The National Academies Press, Washington, DC
5. Kanagalingam MG, Forouhi NG, Greer IA et al (2005) Changes in booking body mass index over a decade: retrospective analysis from a Glasgow maternity hospital. BJOG 112:1431–1433
6. Hedderson MM, Williams MA, Holt VL et al (2008) Body mass index and weight gain prior to pregnancy and risk of gestational diabetes mellitus. Am J Obstet Gynecol 198(4):409. e1–409.e7

7. Sibai BM, Gordon T, Thom E et al (1995) Risk factors for preeclampsia in healthy nulliparous women: a prospective multicenter study. The National Institute of Child Health and Human Development Network of Maternal-Fetal Medicine Units. Am J Obstet Gynecol 172(2Pt1): 642–648

8. Jaarvie E, Ramsay JE (2010) Obstetric management of obesity in pregnancy. Semin Fetal Neonatal Med 15(2):83–88

9. Waller DK, Show GM, Rasmussen SA et al (2007) Prepregnancy obesity as a risk factor for structural birth defects. Arch Pediatr Adolesc Med 161(8):745–750

10. Ehrenberg HM, Mercer BM, Catalano PM (2004) The influence of obesity and diabetes on the prevalence of macrosomia. Am J Obstet Gynecol 191(3):964–968

11. Davies GAL, Maxwell C, Mc Leod L (2010) SOGC clinical practice guideline obesity in pregnancy No.239. Int J Gynaecol Obstet 110(2):167–173

12. CMACE/RCOG (2010) Joint guideline. Management of women with obesity in pregnancy. Published on march 2010. Available on: www.rcog.org.uk/globalassets/documents/guidelines/ cmacercogjointguidelinemanagementwomenobesitypregnancya.pdf

13. Lewis G, Confidential Enquiry into Maternal and Child Healths (2007) Saving mother's lives-reviewing maternal deaths to make motherhood safer 2003–2005. CEMACH, London

14. Lumley J, Watson L, Watson M et al (2001) Periconceptional supplementation with folate and/ or multivitamins for preventing neural tube defect. Cochrane Database of Syst Rev (3):CD001056

15. NICE (2014) Diabetes in pregnancy guidelines update. NICE (2015). Diabetes in pregnancy: management from preconception to the postnatal period. Published on 25 February 2015. Available on: www.nice.org.uk/guidance/ng3

16. merican College of Obstetricians and Gynecologists (2013) ACOG committee opinion no. 549: obesity in pregnancy. Obstet Gynecol 121:213–217

17. ISS-LG Ministero della Salute (2011) Gravidanza Fisiologica, linee guida. Available on: www. snlg-iss.it/cms/files/LG_Gravidanza.pdf

18. Rasmussen SA, Chu SY, Kim SY et al (2008) Maternal obesity and risk of neural tube defect: a metaanalysis. Am J Obstet Gynecol 198:611–619

19. Leddy MA, Power ML, Schulkin JS (2008) The impact of maternal obesity on maternal and fetal health. Rev Obstet Gynecol 1:170–178

20. Conferenza nazionale di Consenso per Raccomandazione ed Implementazione delle nuove linee guida per lo screening e la diagnosi del diabete gestazionale (GDM). 27 Mar 2010. sidi-talia@siditalia.it

21. RCOG (2009) Clinical green top guidelines no 37. RCOG (2015). Reducing the Risk of Venous Thromboembolism during Pregnancy and the Puerperium. Green-top Guideline No. 37a. Published on April 2015. Available on: www.rcog.org.uk/globalassets/documents/guide-lines/gtg-37a.pdf

22. Istituto Nazionale di Ricerca per gli Alimenti e la Nutrizione (INRAN) (2006) Linee guida per una alimentazione italiana. http://www.inran.it/servizi_cittadino/stare_bene/guida_corretta_ alimentazione

23. Institute of Medicine, National Academy of Sciences, Food and Nutrition Board (1990) Nutrition during pregnancy. National Academy, Washington DC

24. Position of the American Dietetic Association (2002) Nutrition and lifestyle for a healthy preg-nancy outcome. J Am Diet Assoc 102:1479–1490

25. Mottola M, Giroux I, Gratton R et al (2010) Nutritional exercise prevent excess weight gain in overweight pregnant women. Med Sci Sports Exerc 42:265–272

26. AGOG (2009) Practice bulletin 105 bariatric surgery and pregnancy. Obstet Gynecol 113(6):1405–1413

Childhood Obesity

10

Claudio Maffeis, Maria Rosaria Licenziati, Andrea Vania,
Piernicola Garofalo, Giuseppe Di Mauro, Margherita Caroli,
Giuseppe Morino, Paolo Siani, and Giampietro Chiamenti

C. Maffeis (✉)
Unit of Pediatric Diabetes and Metabolic Disorders, University Hospital of Verona,
Indian Society of Pediatrics,
Verona, Italy
e-mail: claudio.maffeis@univr.it

M.R. Licenziati
Unit of Auxology and Endocrinology, Department of Pediatrics,
AORN Santobono-Pausilipon, Italian Society of Endocrinology and Pediatric Diabetology,
Naples, Italy

A. Vania
Centre for Paediatric Dietetics and nutrition, Department of Paediatrics,
"Sapienta" University, Italian Society of Pediatric Nutrition, Rome, Italy

P. Garofalo
Endocrine Unit, Villa Sofia-Cervello Hospital, Italian Society of Adolescent Medicine,
Palermo, Italy

G. Di Mauro
Health Search Institute, Italian Pediatric Society – Prevention and Social, Florence, Italy

M. Caroli
Nutrition Unit, Department of Prevention, Italian Society of Obesity, Brindisi, Italy

G. Morino
Bambin Gesù Children's Hospital, Italian Association of Clinical Dietetics and Nutrition,
Rome, Italy

P. Siani
Medical Genetics and Pediatric unit, Department of Pediatrics, AORN Santobono-Pausilipon,
Cultural Association of Pediatricians, Naples, Italy

G. Chiamenti
Community Pediatrician, Italian Federation of Pediatricians, Verona, Italy

© Springer International Publishing Switzerland 2016
P. Sbraccia et al. (eds.), *Clinical Management of Overweight and Obesity:
Recommendations of the Italian Society of Obesity (SIO)*,
DOI 10.1007/978-3-319-24532-4_10

10.1 Introduction

There is a high prevalence of obesity among children, which has shown a steady increase in recent decades, despite some recent signs of stabilization in many industrialized countries, including Italy. The obese child frequently presents metabolic and nonmetabolic risk factors, often manifesting overt morbidity for hypertension, dyslipidemia, glucose intolerance, eating disorders, among others, and a life expectancy lower than that of nonobese children. In addition, the onset of obesity in childhood tends to persist (40–80 % chance) into adulthood. These findings suggest the importance and urgency to identify precociously overweight and obesity in childhood, to treat overweight and its complications, and to implement preventive measures in the general population and especially in those at greatest risk.

This document represents the consensus of a group of pediatric experts on the subject, delegates from scientific societies, and organizations of pediatricians and is intended as an updated tool, quick and practical on the issue of obesity in childhood and adolescence.

10.2 Diagnosis

When evaluating an overweight child, it is always necessary to exclude, using the child's medical history and a thorough objective examination, a secondary cause from endocrine disorders, congenital or acquired hypothalamic alterations, genetic syndromes, and use of drugs.

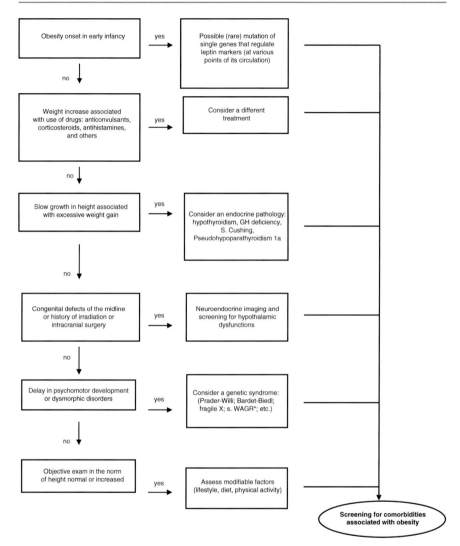

Recommended assessments in cases of childhood obesity (*WAGR=t. di Wilms +aniridia+genitourinary alterations+mental retardation) (From Han et al. [24])

10.2.1 Clinical Diagnosis

- *Babies up to 24 months*: a diagnosis of obesity is based on a weight/length ratio (2006 OMS reference tables) with cut-off values of:
  Risk of overweight: >85th percentile (>1 DS)
  Overweight: >97th percentile (>2 DS)
  Obese: >99th percentile (>3 DS). (*Level of evidence*: VI, *Strength of recommendation*: A)
- *Children between 24 months and 18 years*: a diagnosis of obesity is based on the body mass index (BMI): weight (kg)/height (m²).

Reference Tables
- OMS 2006 for children between two and five years of age, with the following cut-offs: weight to length ratio/BMI >85th P (>1 DS) – "risk of overweight"; >97th P (>2 DS) – "overweight"; >99th P (>3 DS) – "obese"
- OMS 2007 tables after five years of age, with the following cut-offs:
- BMI >85th P (>1 DS) – "overweight"; >97th P (>2 DS) – "obese" [Note]
- BMI SIEDP tables between 2 and 18 years. Overweight: BMI >75th P (which corresponds to the percentile that intersects a BMI of 25 at the age of 18 years); obesity: BMI >95th P (which corresponds to the percentile that intersects a BMI of 30 at the age of 18 years). (*Level of evidence*: VI, *Strength of recommendation*: A)

We stress the fact that children in this category require careful anthropometric monitoring and nutritional supervision/education.

Given the strong association between body fat distribution and metabolic complications, it is helpful to calculate in all children with excess weight from the age of five years and upwards the relationship between waist circumference and height. A value greater than 0.5 regardless of gender, age, and ethnicity is associated with an increase in cardiovascular risk factors, regardless of BMI. (*Level of evidence*: I, *Strength of recommendation*: A)

- In the case of "overweight," it is also helpful to take a precise measurement of a triceps skinfold in order to avoid false positives and/or negatives (reference tables: Barlow & Dietz). Cut-off values: 85th percentile for "overweight," 95th percentile for "obesity." (*Level of evidence*: I, *Strength of recommendation*: B)

10.3 Complications

In cases of frequent morbidity in the obese child, it is recommended to look into metabolic and nonmetabolic complications. This should also be done for the overweight child with a family history of cardiovascular risk factors (hypertension, diabetes, dyslipidemia, cardiovascular disease). (*Level of evidence*: I, *Strength of recommendation*: A)

The most important organic complications are dyslipidemia, hypertension, nonalcoholic fatty liver disease, steatohepatitis, glucose intolerance, polycystic ovaries, orthopedic and respiratory complications. The most frequent psychological complications are disorders concerning body image, eating habits, and depression. (*Level of evidence: I, Strength of recommendation: A*)

To assess the risks of endocrine-metabolic complications

- Lab tests advised: glucose, lipid profile, and transaminases. (*Level of evidence: I, Strength of recommendation: A*), for insulinemia: (*Level of evidence: VI, Strength of recommendation: C*)
- The load curve for the diagnosis of IGT or T2D should be reserved for patients with fasting blood glucose >100 mg/dl or a family history of T2D or in the presence of acanthosis nigricans, polycystic ovary syndrome (PCOS), or metabolic syndrome. The load curve is also helpful in overweight children with at least two risk criteria such as ethnicity, family history of type 2 diabetes, acanthosis nigricans, PCOS, and metabolic syndrome. (*Level of evidence: VI, Strength of recommendation: A*)

  Screening for diagnosis of metabolic syndrome: it is advisable to make the diagnosis in the presence of at least three of the following situations: BMI suggestive of obesity or waist circumference/height ratio >0.5, systolic and/or diastolic blood pressure >95th percentile, fasting blood glucose >100 mg/dl, triglycerides >95th percentile, HDL cholesterol <5th percentile (reference tables SINUPE: Consensus Conference of the Italian Society of Pediatrics on Childhood and Adolescent Obesity, 2006).[1] (*Level of evidence: I, Strength of recommendation: A*)
- Pelvic ultrasound and hormonal doses in cases of suspected PCOS. (*Level of evidence: I, Strength of recommendation: A*)

10.3.1 Assessing the Risk of Cardiovascular Complications

- Blood pressure measurement (reference tables of the National High Blood Pressure Education Program Working Group on High Blood Pressure in Children and Adolescents, Pediatrics 2004).
- Hypertension is defined by the presence of SBP and/or DBP >95th percentile for age, gender, and height, measured on at least three occasions.
- In patients where hypertension is confirmed, more thorough diagnostic tests should be done: an examination by a cardiac specialist with ECG and echocardiogram, standard urinalysis, microalbuminuria, creatinine and potassium levels. (*Level of evidence: I, Strength of recommendation: A*)[1]

---

[1] The waist circumference/height ratio, with a cut-off ≥0.5, is a marker of cardiovascular risk even in children. There are no age- and sex-specific reference tables for the Italian population. There is currently no shared and accepted definition of metabolic syndrome in children and adolescents.

10.3.2 Assessing the Risk of Nonalcoholic Fatty Liver Disease or Steatohepatitis

Liver ultrasound is recommended for all obese children and adolescents. In children with confirmed ALT >40 IU/L or palpable liver, more thorough diagnostic tests are advisable with gamma-GT and differential diagnosis of hepatitis.

10.3.3 Mental Health Assessment

Stressing the importance of an assessment of the psychological component of obesity, it is important to select subjects with a family history of eating or psychiatric disorders or subjects who make the clinician suspect the presence of DCA or psychological disorder during the medical examination. These children/teenagers should therefore undergo psychological counseling-psychiatric evaluation to identify the cognitive and emotional determinants, the patients' relational context, and diagnosis of DCA. (*Level of evidence*: V, *Strength of recommendation*: A)

10.4 The Setting for Care

For the prevention and treatment of child/adolescent obesity, it is important to set up a pediatric network that offers a continuum of care from birth to late adolescence. The objectives of the network are the ubiquity of treatment of obesity in all the geographical areas of relevance, ensuring that all patients are treated at the appropriate level, according to different clinical situations.

The network is structured on three levels:

Level one: the pediatrician. This provides the first level of care to children and plays an important role in the prevention and treatment of obesity in children.

Level two: out-patient services where families can consult with a pediatrician who has documented experience in obesity and who works in interdisciplinary teams with dietitians, nutritionists, psychologists, and, possibly, an educator with a degree in physical education. Access to these services is based on referral from the pediatrician.

Level three: a specialist center for the diagnosis and treatment of obesity (at least one center per region or county). It should be organized on a multidisciplinary basis, involving different professionals: pediatric experts on childhood obesity, clinical nutritionists, endocrinologists, psychologists, dietitians, nurses, trained physical education personnel, and physiotherapists. The specialist center for the diagnosis and treatment refers a patient to a clinical department (usually operative complex units of pediatrics/pediatric clinic) with facilities for genetic analysis, imaging, functional tests, expert advice, activities of bariatric surgery, etc., and has the task of handling complicated cases of obesity, also admitting patients to day hospital or inpatient facilities. The center has also the role of coordinating the activities of the network by providing training for the members of the network and coordinating research activities.

The second and third levels work together in a coordinated manner by communicating the treatment path chosen to the PLS, all their results, and the program of therapy and follow-up. (*Level of evidence*: *VI, Strength of recommendation*: *A*)

10.5 Treatment

10.5.1 Objectives

The primary purpose of treating obesity is the long-term improvement of physical health through healthy lifestyles. This in itself improves the weight in a proportion of patients; in others, it is necessary to introduce additional behavioral modification strategies to promote a negative energy balance. To do this, we need the active involvement of the entire family. (*Level of evidence*: *I, Strength of recommendation*: *A*)

If there are complications of obesity, their resolution or at least their treatment is a priority objective. (*Level of evidence*: *VI, Strength of recommendation*: *A*)

Psychological health (self-esteem, correct attitudes toward food and one's body) and the improvement of quality of life are also crucial in the treatment goals. (*Level of evidence*: *I, Strength of recommendation*: *A*)

In all children or adolescents with excess weight, but without complications, a reduction of the level of overweight is the most important target. That does not necessarily mean a loss of weight. In fact, in the case the weight is kept constant, the physiologic increase of height with age promotes a reduction of BMI, possibly to obtain a return to a BMI in the normal range. (*Level of evidence*: *VI, Strength of recommendation*: *A*)

In all children or adolescents with excess weight and complications, it is necessary to strive for resolution or at least improve the complications mainly through weight loss, and possibly to obtain a return to a BMI in the normal range. (*Level of evidence*: *VI, Strength of recommendation*: *A*)

The therapeutic process must provide for the taking charge of the subject by a specialist center and provide a multidisciplinary plan to change eating habits and lifestyles by setting simple goals that can be modified at any time.

Frequency of check-ups: These should be scheduled monthly and at intervals not exceeding two months.[2] (*Level of evidence*: *I, Strength of recommendation*: *A*)

---

[2] Recent data indicate that an efficient treatment plan means that time spent globally with a professional for at least one year should not be less than 25 h.

"Therapeutic education" (OMS 1998) provides an educational process to improve choices related to nutrition and physical activity. This involves a preliminary critical assessment of the eating habits of the whole family through a thorough history (composition of meals, frequency and mode of intake of foods, food preferences, leisure time, time spent looking at a screen, use of the car to get around, etc.), with particular focus on the seasonings used, cooking methods and portions. It is also wise to use a diary to keep a record of eating habits and physical activity — kept by the patient and/or parents (or caregivers of the child) — for up to 3–7 days to be evaluated by a pediatrician and/or a dietitian. (*Level of evidence*: *VI, Strength of recommendation*: *A*)

10.6   Nutrition

One goal is to divide the daily calorie intake into at least five meals over the day (three meals + two snacks). (*Level of evidence*: *I, Strength of recommendation*: *A*)

An adequate breakfast in the morning is highly recommended. (*Level of evidence*: *I, Strength of recommendation*: *A*)

The use of diets in general, especially if unbalanced (high protein and low carbohydrate) or one that contains very few calories, is strongly discouraged. Very low calorie diets may be prescribed only in special cases and under close clinical monitoring (specialist center at the third level). (*Level of evidence*: *VI, Strength of recommendation*: *A*)

The suggested way to limit calorie intake is to restrict or replace specific high-calorie foods with others less rich in calories. (*Level of evidence*: *VI, Strength of recommendation*: *A*)

The total protein content must comply with the LARN recommendations for sex, age, and ideal weight for height. It is suggested that the 14 meals per week have the following frequencies of use: meat, three to four times a week; fish, three to four times a week; legumes, three to four times a week; cheese and eggs, once a week. (*Level of evidence*: *VI, Strength of recommendation*: *A*)

Carbohydrates should account for at least 50 % of total calories, preferring low glycemic index foods (cereals such as pasta, barley, and whole wheat products, which should be consumed twice a day; legumes; fruit and vegetables in season, not canned or pureed, which should make up five servings a day) and by limiting foods that combine a high glycemic index to a high glycemic load (bread, rice, potatoes, sweets, sugar, fruit juices, sweet drinks). (*Level of evidence*: *VI, Strength of recommendation*: *A*)

The total fat in the diet should account for no more than 30 % of total calories. (*Level of evidence*: *I, Strength of recommendation*: *A*)

The adequate intake of fiber in grams/day should be between the age of the child +5 and the child's age +10. Five servings a day of fruits and vegetables in season, not canned or pureed, and legumes four times a week are recommended. (*Level of evidence*: *VI, Strength of recommendation*: *A*)

10.7   Physical Activity

Motivate parents to a more active lifestyle. (*Level of evidence*: *I*, *Strength of recommendation*: *A*)

Program the reduction of time spent doing sedentary activities, in particular the time spent with video displays (TV, computer, video games). (*Level of evidence*: *I*, *Strength of recommendation*: *A*)

Promote active play, possibly outdoors and in groups.

Promote the participation in regular organized sport activity, something the child likes, something fun, and where the main goal is not competition but physical activity adapted to the clinical conditions and obesity level of the child. (*Level of evidence*: *VI*, *Strength of recommendation*: *A*)

The intensity of the exercise planned should be moderate at first (or not to exceed 65 % of maximal heart rate or 55 % of VO_2 max). (*Level of evidence*: *VI*, *Strength of recommendation*: *A*)

Some type of aerobic exercise (swimming, cycling, walking) is recommended to be practiced daily. You can also combine exercises that stimulate flexibility and strength, especially of the arms and trunk, which are age appropriate and adequate for the stage of development of the child, with a frequency of two to three times a week. (*Level of evidence*: *I*, *Strength of recommendation*: *A*)

The duration of the exercise should be 30 min initially and can be increased gradually in subsequent sessions. (*Level of evidence*: *VI*, *Strength of recommendation*: *A*)

10.8   Cognitive Behavioral Approach

As part of a course of treatment, it may be useful to have a systemic cognitive behavioral approach only in the family up to the age of 8–10 years and mostly limited to the family thereafter. (*Level of evidence*: *I*, *Strength of recommendation*: *B*)

The techniques considered to be most helpful in the treatment of an obese child over ten years old are: keeping a food diary (self-monitoring), keeping a diary of physical activity or the use of a pedometer, preparation for any contingency, control of stimuli, cognitive restructuring, and positive reinforcement. (*Level of evidence*: *VI*, *Strength of recommendation*: *B*)

The use of this approach to treatment requires special training of the professionals involved and the collaboration of a psychologist. (*Level of evidence*: *VI*, *Strength of recommendation*: *A*)

10.9   Drug Therapy for Obesity

The use of drugs in the treatment of childhood obesity should be considered only in cases of very severe forms of obesity that do not respond to modifications of diet and cognitive behavioral therapy. This could cause complications that could potentially be irreversible.

The use of medicines in children can be expected only in the context of controlled clinical trials.

The drug used for children is orlistat, the effectiveness of which (always in combination with diet and exercise), however, is modest. The Food and Drug Administration has approved the use of orlistat for patients over the age of 12 years.

The use of metformin is recommended in cases of obese children or adolescents with T2DM. (*Level of evidence*: *VI, Strength of recommendation*: *A*)

10.10 Bariatric Surgery

Pediatric bariatric surgery is considered a last resort in patients resistant to all other treatments, especially if you are in the presence of life-threatening complications. Please refer to the chapter on "Bariatric Surgery" (see Chap. 6).

10.11 Prevention

Prevention is the best cost/benefit approach for the management of obesity in children and, in the future, of adulthood. Obesity is a multifactorial disease, so preventive measures should be implemented on all the causes of aggravation and children should be treated from birth, especially if there is a family history of obesity or diabetes or if the baby was born small for gestational age.

10.11.1 Primary Prevention

The most important figure involved in primary prevention is the family pediatrician. Most of the recommendations below are based on the results of observational cohort studies or cross-sectional studies that reported a frequent, significant association (direct or indirect) between a specific behavior and the current or future risk of overweight (Levels of evidence IV), with the weakness of not being able to establish with certainty the exact causality involved in these associations. There is a need for more randomized controlled trials to better define the real impact of a given behavior on the development or aggravation of excess weight.

The urgent need to combat the current obesity epidemic underway leads us, however, for ethical reasons, to promote preventive measures based on the best evidence available at the time rather than wait inopportunely for the best evidence possible. Therefore, on the basis of this line of thinking, the recommended preventive actions are:

- Encourage and support breastfeeding for as long as possible; support limited complementary feeding (weaning) to protein, especially from animals. (*Level of evidence I, Strength of recommendation*: *A*)

- Encourage an adequate amount of sleep from the first year of life. (*Level of evidence*: *VI*, *Strength of evidence*: *B*)
- Avoid using food as a reward or punishment or to calm restlessness regardless of the need to eat. (*Level of evidence*: *VI*, *Strength of recommendation*: *A*)
- Have an adequate breakfast regularly in the morning. (*Level of evidence*: *I*, *Strength of recommendation*: *A*)
- Have as many family meals as possible, possibly with the parents. (*Level of evidence*: *I*, *Strength of recommendation*: *A*)
- Limit the intake of high-calorie foods. (*Level of evidence*: *I*, *Strength of recommendation*: *A*)
- Teach the child to satisfy his thirst by drinking water and not sweetened beverages. (*Level of evidence*: *VI*, *Strength of recommendation*: *A*)
- Avoid using fruit juices as a substitute for fruit. (*Level of evidence*: *VI*, *Strength of recommendation*: *A*)
- Increase the amount of fruit, vegetables, and legumes in the usual family meals (it is recommended to consume five servings a day of fruits and vegetables and legumes three to four times a week). (*Level of evidence*: *VI*, *Strength of recommendation*: *A*)
- Provide a balanced diet in terms of macronutrients, including adequate fiber and calcium. (*Level of evidence*: *VI*, *Strength of recommendation*: *A*)
- Guarantee that the energy provided by lipids, carbohydrates, and proteins is in age-appropriate amounts. (*Level of evidence*: *VI*, *Strength of recommendation*: *A*)
- Limit the total time spent watching TV, using the computer, and playing video games; total time should not exceed more than 2 h a day after the age of two years, selecting quality programs and avoiding exposure to video screens for children under the age of two years. (*Level of evidence*: *I*, *Strength of recommendation*: *A*)
- Turn off the TV during meals and do not allow a TV or computer in the children's bedroom. (*Level of evidence*: *I*, *Strength of recommendation*: *A*)
- Encourage active play outdoors as much as possible. (*Level of evidence*: *VI*, *Strength of recommendation*: *A*)
- Find ways for the whole family to get physical exercise every day: encourage walking instead of depending on the car and encourage the practice of sports the children enjoy. A child of normal weight should get at least 60 min of moderate-intense physical exercise a day (the minutes can be distributed throughout the day). (*Level of evidence*: *VI*, *Strength of recommendation*: *A*)

10.11.2 Aimed Prevention

Criteria for identifying individuals at increased risk

- Mother and/or father with BMI >25 kg/m^2 and/or with a history of cardiometabolic complications or low socioeconomic status. (*Level of evidence*: *I*, *Strength of recommendation*: *A*)

- Birth weight: large (LGA) or small for gestational age (SGA). (*Level of evidence*: *I*, *Strength of recommendation*: *A*)
- Excessive speed of weight gain in the first two years of life (>1 SD on the WHO reference table for the weight/length ratio according to the 2006 WHO curves). (*Level of evidence*: *I*, *Strength of recommendation*: *A*)
- Early adiposity rebound: early upward turn of the BMI trajectory between two and five years. (*Level of evidence*: *I*, *Strength of recommendation*: *A*)
- Subjects with a weight/length ratio in the "overweight risk" ranging between the 85th and 97th percentiles of the 2006 WHO curves. (*Level of evidence*: *III*, *Strength of recommendation*: *A*)
- Sociocultural disadvantages associated with one or more of the above: in underprivileged neighborhoods with strong social unrest, the pediatrician should be concerned with implementing community policies (contacting schools and other organizations in the area—parishes or other church communities and other places where people meet) rather than focusing on the individual, to ensure that these interventions actually have an effect on the health of the child in treatment. (*Level of evidence*: *III*, *Strength of recommendation*: *A*)

  In addition to specific actions taken within the family, in schools and in the healthcare environment, it is fundamental to set up a universal preventive approach, whose responsibility falls to the local political administration in collaboration with scientific/medical associations. To ensure that the measures taken are effective in the long term, it is important that they are integrated and coordinated at both regional and national levels. It is not likely that the obesity problem will be solved except through actions taken in the social as well as physical environments in which people live. (*Level of evidence*: *VI*, *Strength of recommendation*: *A*)

10.12 Teenagers with Obesity

Treating adolescent obesity is a challenge for both the family doctor and the specialist because of the dramatic changes in the cognitive, neurochemical, and psychosocial characteristics of young people of this age. Obesity in adolescence has a very high risk of persistence, aggravation, and onset of comorbidities; therefore, it is necessary to set up specific programs that are pleasant and nonrestrictive.

The therapeutic programs for teenagers cannot be entrusted exclusively to the family as in the case of children; the teenagers have the right and duty to participate and to be treated with appropriate therapy plans adapted to their degree of maturity and responsibility.

The principle of *health gain*, that is, making healthy choices easy, at this age is extremely beneficial and requested by the teenagers themselves. Adolescents are often not aware of their problem or do not know how to quantify it properly. We need to make them aware without creating derision and help them follow a path of healthy and feasible changes without the risk of developing a more serious condition.

Overweight/obesity and eating disorders are the two major public health problems concerning this age. Today the ascertained risk factors for eating disorders are: frequent dieting, critical comments about one's weight, body and eating habits, frequenting environments that emphasize being thin. All these factors are found in adolescents who suffer from excess weight. These facts, although statistics are still low, underline the need for preventive measures and treatment of obesity in adolescence with new models that take into account both the risks associated with obesity and those related to eating disorders.

It is not easy to get an adolescent to take an active part in lengthy health treatments and those involving a team of experts. The characteristics of adolescence (a desire for independence, the attitude to challenge authority, and improper behavior) make the therapeutic approach difficult. Obesity is seen as a disability, something to be ashamed of that causes one not to be accepted by others. The characteristic refusal to follow imposed rules, the inability to have a balanced assessment of the "risk," the need for immediate and visible results, the desire to be accepted and appreciated by one's peers, the importance of body image, and sensitivity to derision are fundamental and inalienable priorities.

10.12.1 Particulars of the Approach regarding Adolescents

- Give a primary role to the adolescent in his particular treatment program and facilitate his internal motivation, not to mention the role of the entire family.
- Develop a multicomponent project (healthier diet modeled on the Mediterranean diet; reduction of physical inactivity by offering pleasing alternatives to television, electronic games, computers, and smartphones; increased physical exercise or age-appropriate games; healthy sleep; and less stress).
- Use an approach based on interviews that motivate (Janicke 2014), with a team of professionals (physician-psychologist-dietician) who work closely together in the most serious cases—experts that have experience with this age group.
- Reduce intrafamily conflicts and promote healthy role models on the part of the parents and grandparents, encouraging a situation that favors the gradual autonomy of the teens, instead of prescribing and imposing restrictive diets.
- Shift the goal of treatment from body weight to global health so that the teens can fully meet their life objectives.

Bibliography

1. A collaborative statement from Dieticians of Canada, Canadian Paediatric Society, The College of Family Physicians, and Community Health Nurses of Canada (2010) A health professional's guide for using the new WHO growth charts. Paediatr Child Health 15:84–90
2. Alhassan S, Sirard JR et al (2007) The effect of increasing outdoor play time on physical activity in Latino preschool children. Int J Pediatr Obes 2(3):153–158
3. American Academy of Pediatrics, American Public Health Association, National Resource Center for Health and Safety in Child Care and Early Education 2010. Preventing Childhood

Obesity in Early care and Education Programs; selected standards from Caring for Our Children: National Health and Safety Performance Standards 3rd Edition 2011

4. American Academy of Pediatrics-Committee on Nutrition (2001) The use and misuse of fruit juices in children. Pediatrics 107:1210–1213

5. Ambruzzi MA, G (2010) Valerio "Sovrappeso e Obesit. nel bambino da 0 a 6 anni" J Medical Books Edizioni S.r.l. Viareggio (LU)

6. Anzman SL, Rollins BY et al (2010) Parental influence on children's early eating environments and obesity risk: implications for prevention. Int J Obes (Lond) 34:1116–1124

7. Atlantis E, Barnes EH, Fiatarone Singh MA (2006) Efficacy of exercise for treating overweight in children and adolescents: a systematic review. Int J Obes (Lond) 30:1027–1040

8. Barlow SE (2007) Expert committee recommendations regarding the prevention, assessment and treatment of child and adolescent overweight and obesity: summary report. Pediatrics 120:S164–S192

9. Berge JM, Larson N et al (2011) Are parents of young children practicing healthy nutrition and physical activity behaviors? Pediatrics 127:881–887

10. Burdette HL, Whitaker RC (2005) Resurrecting free play in young children. Arch Pediatr Adolesc Med 159:46–50

11. Center for Disease Control and Prevention (2010) Use of the World Health Organization and CDC growth charts for children aged 0–59 months in the United States. Recommendations and Reports 2010: <charts>

12. Cole TJ, Lobstein T (2012) Extended internation (IOTF) body mass index cut-offd for thinness, overweight and obesity. Pediatr Obes 7:284–294

13. Cole TJ, Faith MS, Pietrobelli A, Heo M (2005) What is the best measure of adiposity change in growing children: BMI, BMI%, BMI z-score or BMI centile? Eur J Clin Nutr 59:419–425

14. Cortese S, Falissard B, Pigaiani Y, Banzato C, Bogoni G, Pellegrino M, Vincenzi B, Angriman M, Cook S, Purper-Ouakil D, Dalla Bernardina B, Maffeis C (2010) The relationship between body mass index and body size dissatisfaction in young adolescents: spline function analysis. J Am Diet Assoc 110(7):1098–1102

15. Cortese S, Falissard B, Angriman M, Pigaiani Y, Banzato C, Bogoni G, Pellegrino M, Cook S, Pajno-Ferrara F, Bernardina BD, Mouren MC, Maffeis C (2009) The relationship between body size and depression symptoms in adolescents. J Pediatr 154(1):86–90

16. Council on Communications and Media (2011) Policy statement- children, adolescents, obesity, and the media. Pediatrics 128:201–208

17. De Onis M, Onyango AW et al (2007) Development of a WHO growth reference for school-aged children and adolescents. Bull World Health Organ 85:660–667

18. Dixon H, Scully M et al (2007) The effects of television advertisements for junk food versus nutritious food on chlidren's food attitudes and preferences. Soc Sci Med 65:1311–1323

19. Flegal KM, Ogden CL (2011) Childhood obesity: are we all speaking the same language? Adv Nutr 2:159S–166S

20. Francis LA, Susman EJ (2009) Self -regulation and rapid weight gain in children from age 3 to 12 years. Arch Pediatr Adolesc Med 163(4):297–302

21. Gooze RA, Anderson SE et al (2011) Prolonged bottle use and obesity at 5,5 years of age in US children. J Pediatr 159(3):431–436

22. Griffiths LJ, Hawkins SS et al (2010) Risk factors for rapid weight gain in preschool children: findings from a UK-wide prospective study. Int J Obes (Lond) 34:624–632

23. Hammons AJ, Fiese BH (2011) Is frequency of shared family meals related to the nutrition health of children and adolescents? Pediatrics 127, e000

24. Han JC, Lawlor DA, Kimm SY (2010) Childhood obesity. Lancet 375(9727):1737–1748

25. Haute Autorit. de Sant.. Surpoids et ob.sit. de l'enfant et de l'adolescent. Recommandation de bonne pratique Sept 2011

26. Huh SY, Rifas SL et al (2011) Timing of solid food introduction and risk of obesity in preschool-aged children. Pediatrics 127:e544–e551

27. Iaia M (2009) "Early adiposity rebound": indicatore precoce di rischio per lo sviluppo di obesità e di complicanze metaboliche. Quaderni acp 16(2):72–78

28. IOM Committee on Obesity Prevention Policies for Young Children (2011) Early childhood obesity prevention policies. The National Academies Press, Washington, DC
29. Keller S, Schulz P (2010) Distorted food pyramid in kids programmes: a content analysis of television advertising watched in Switzerland. Eur J Public Health 21:1–6
30. Levy-Marchal C, Arslanian S, Cutfield W, et al. ESPE-LWPES-ISPAD-APPES-APEG-SLEP-JSPE; Insulin Resistance in Children Consensus Conference Group (2010) Insulin resistance in children: consensus, perspective, and future directions. J Clin Endocrinol Metab 95(12):5189–5198
31. Loprinzi P, Trost S (2010) Parental influences on physical activity behaviour in preschool children. Prev Med 50:129–133
32. Maffeis C (2005) Il bambino obeso e le sue complicanze. Dalla conoscenza scientifica alla pratica clinica. SEE Ed. Firenze
33. Maffeis C, Banzato C, Brambilla P, Cerutti F, Corciulo N, Cuccarolo G, Di Pietro M, Franzese A, Gennari M, Balsamo A, Grugni G, Iughetti L, Del Giudice EM, Petri A, Trada M, Yiannakou P, Obesity Study Group of the Italian Society of Pediatric Endocrinology and Diabetology (2010) Insulin resistance is a risk factor for high blood pressure regardless of body size and fat distribution in obese children. Nutr Metab Cardiovasc Dis 20(4):266–273
34. Maffeis C, Banzato C, Rigotti F, Nobili V, Valandro S, Manfredi R, Morandi A (2011) Biochemical parameters and anthropometry predict NAFLD in obese children. J Pediatr Gastroenterol Nutr 53(6):590–593
35. Monteiro PO, Victora CG (2005) Rapid growth in infancy and childhood and obesity in later life- a systematic review. Obes Rev 6:143–154
36. Morandi A, Maschio M, Marigliano M, Miraglia Del Giudice E, Moro B, Peverelli P, Maffeis C (2014) Screening for impaired glucose tolerance in obese children and adolescents: a validation and implementation study. Pediatr Obes 9:17–25. Pearson N, Biddle SJ et al (2008) Family correlates of fruit and vegetable consumption in children and adolescents: a systematic review. Public Health Nutr 12(2):267–283
37. American Diabetes Association. Standards of Medical care in Diabetes (2014). Diabetes care 37(Suppl 1):S14–80
38. Pryor LE, Tremblay RE et al (2011) Developmental trajectories of body mass index in early childhood and their risk factors. An 8 year longitudinal study. Arch Pediatr Adolesc Med 165(10):906–991
39. Regione Emilia Romagna (2010) OKkio alla salute:Risultati dell'indagine 2010: www.okkio-allaallasalute.it
40. Reilly JJ (2008) Physical activity, sedentary behaviour and energy balance in the preschool child: opportunities for early obesity prevention. Proc Nutr Soc 67:317–325
41. Reilly JJ, Armstrong J, Dorosty AR et al (2005) Early life risk factors for obesity in childhood: cohort study. BMJ 330:1357–1364
42. Rolland Cachera MF, Deheeger M, Maillot M et al (2006) Early adiposity rebound: causes and consequences for obesity in children and adults. Int J Obes (Lond) 30:S11–S17
43. Societ (2001) Italiana di Nutrizione Pediatrica. Terapia dietetica dell'obesit. essenziale. Riv Ital Ped (IJP) 27:275:279
44. Societ. Italiana di Pediatria. Obesit. del bambino e dell'adolescente: consensus su prevenzione, diagnosi e terapia. Istituto Scotti Bassani per la ricerca e l'informazione scientifica e nutrizionale, Milano 2006 (I Ed.)
45. Spill M, Birch L et al (2010) Eating vegetables first: the use of portion size to increase vegetable intake in preschool children. Am J Clin Nutr 91:1237–1243
46. Strasburger V, Jordan A et al (2010) Health effects of media on children and adolescents. Pediatrics 125:756–767
47. Tandon P, Zhou C et al (2011) Preschoolers' total daily screen time at home and by type of Child Care. J Pediatr 158:297–300
48. Taveras E, Gortmaker S (2011) Randomized controlled trial to improve primary care to prevent and manage childhood obesity. The high five for kids study. Arch Pediatr Adolesc Med. Published on line 4 Apr 2011. www.archpediatrics.com

49. Taveras EM, Rifas SL et al (2008) Short sleep duration in infancy and risk of childhood over-weight. Arch Pediatr Adolesc Med 162:305–311
50. Taveras EM, Rifas-Shiman SL, Belfort MB et al (2009) Weight status in the first 6 months of life and obesity at 3 years of age. Pediatrics 123:1177–1183
51. Tucker P (2008) The physical activity levels of preschool-aged children: a systematic review. Early Child Res Q 23:547–558
52. Tucker P, Zandvort M (2011) The influence of parents and the home environment on pre-schoolers' physical activity behaviours: a qualitative investigation of childcare providers' per-spective. BMC Public Health 11:168
53. United States Department of Agricolture, Department of Health and Human Services (2010 Dietary Guidelines for Americans), 7th edition
54. Preventive Services Task Force US (2010) Screening for obesity in children and adolescents: US Preventive Services Task Force Recommendation Statement. Pediatrics 125:361–367
55. VanDijk CE, Innis SM (2009) Growth-curve standards and the assessment of early excess weight gain in infancy. Pediatrics 123:102–108
56. Weiss R, Dziura J, Burgert TS, Tamborlane WV, Taksali SE, Yeckel CW, Allen K, Lopes M, Savoye M, Morrison J, Sherwin RS, Caprio S (2004) Obesity and the metabolic Syndrome in children and adolescents. N Engl J Med 350:2362–2374
57. Whitlock EP, O'Connor EA, Williams SB (2010) Effectiveness of weight management inter-ventions in children: a targeted systematic review for the USPSTF. Pediatrics 125:e396–e418
58. World Health Organization (2001) Infant and young child nutrition. Fiftyfourth World Health Assembly, Geneva, p 54.2
59. World Health Organization (2002) Report of a joint WHO/FAO expert consultation. Diet and nutrition and the prevention of chronic diseases, vol 916, Who technical Report Series. WHO, Geneva
60. World Health Organization. Multicentre Growth Reference Study Group (2006) WHO Child growth standards based on length/height, weight and age. Acta Paediatr 450(suppl):76–85
61. World health Organzation. Growth reference (5–19 years). http://www.who.int/growthref/who2007_bmi_for_age/en/
62. World Health Organization (2008) Training course on child growth assessment. WHO Child growth standards, Geneva. www.who.int/childgrowth/en/index.htlm
63. Wright CM, Emmet PM et al (2010) Tracking of obesity and body fatness through midchild-hood. Arch Dis Child 95:612–617
64. Zecevic C, Tremblay L et al (2010) Parental influence on young children's physical activity. Int J Pediatr. doi:10.1155/2010/468526
65. Zimmerman F, Christakis D et al (2007) Television and DVD/Video viewing in children younger than 2 years. Arch Pediatr Adolesc Med 161:473–479
66. Tirosh A, Shai I, Afek A, Dubnov-Raz G, Ayalon N, Gordon B, Derazne E, Tzur D, Shamis A, Vinker S, Rudich A (2011) Adolescent BMI trajectory and risk of diabetes versus coronary disease. N Engl J Med 364(14):1315–1325
67. Ludwig DS (2012) Weight loss strategies for adolescents: a 14-year-old struggling to lose weight. JAMA 307:498–508
68. Lobstein T, Baur L, Uauy R, for the IASO (2004) Obesity in children and young people: a crisis in public health. Obes Rev 5(Suppl 1):4–104
69. Young S (2014) Healthy behavior change in practical settings. Perm J 18(4):89–92
70. Dietz WH, Baur LA, Hall K, Puhl RM, Taveras EM, Uauy R, Kopelman P (2015) Management of obesity: improvement of health-care training and systems for prevention and care. Lancet 385(9986):2521–2533
71. Rees RW, Caird J, Dickson K, Vigurs C, Thomas J (2014) 'It's on your conscience all the time': a systematic review of qualitative studies examining views on obesity among young people aged 12–18 years in the UK. BMJ Open 4(4):e004404
72. Smith E, Sweeting H, Wright C (2013) 'Do I care ?' Young adults' recalled experiences of early adolescent overweight and obesity: a qualitative study. Int J Obes (Lond) 37(2):303–308

73. Neumark-Sztainer D, Wall M, Guo J, Story M, Haines J, Eisenberg M (2006) Obesity, disordered eating, and eating disorders in a longitudinal study of adolescents: How do dieters fare five years later? J Am Diet Assoc 106:559–568
74. Neumark-Sztainer D, Wall M, Haines J, Story M, Eisenberg ME (2007) Why does dieting predict weight gain in adolescents? Findings from project EAT-II: a 5-year longitudinal study. J Am Diet Assoc 107(3):448–455
75. Neumark-Sztainer DR, Wall MM, Haines JI, Story MT, Sherwood NE, van den Berg PA (2007) Shared risk and protective factors for overweight and disordered eating in adolescents. Am J Prev Med 33:359–369
76. Field AE, Austin SB, Taylor CB, Malspeis S, Rosner B, Rockett HR, Gillman MW, Colditz GA (2003) Relation between dieting and weight change among preadolescents and adolescents. Pediatrics 112:900–906
77. Babio N, Canals J, Pietrobelli A, Pérez S, Arija V (2009) A two-phase population study: relationships between overweight, body composition and risk of eating disorders. Nutr Hosp 24(4):485–491
78. Linee Guida Regionali per la diagnosi ed il trattamento dei disturbi alimentari (2013) Edizione Regione Umbria

Geriatric Obesity

11

Mauro Zamboni, Elena Zoico, Simona Budui,
and Gloria Mazzali

Obesity and fat distribution in older age is associated with a higher risk of comorbidities, cardiovascular disease (CVD) and disability (Levels of evidence II, Classes of recommendations B).

Obesity has functional implications in older individuals and exacerbates the age-related decline in physical function (Levels of evidence II, Classes of recommendations B).

Weight loss improves metabolic and functional outcomes in the elderly (Levels of evidence I, Classes of recommendations A).

Lifestyle changes in older people, with moderate caloric restriction and regular physical exercise, are the recommended therapeutic strategy in older individuals. Physical exercise alone does not determine a significant weight loss in the elderly. (Levels of evidence I, Classes of recommendations A).

Caloric restriction should be moderated in the elderly (not more than 500 kcal/die), and the diet should have an adequate quantity of proteins, calcium, and vitamin D. Older individuals should avoid strongly hypocaloric diets (Levels of evidence II, Classes of recommendations D).

11.1 Prevalence of Obesity in the Elderly

Epidemic obesity is an emerging problem even in the elderly. Obesity prevalence in Americans aged 60 years and older increased from 23.6 % in 1990 to 37.4 % in 2010 [1], while 9.9 % of subjects older than 85 years were obese [2]. Moreover, in the USA from 1999 to 2000 to 2011–2012 the mean waist circumference increased

M. Zamboni (✉) • E. Zoico • S. Budui • G. Mazzali
Department of Medicine, Geriatric Section, University of Verona, Verona, Italy
e-mail: mauro.zamboni@univr.it

© Springer International Publishing Switzerland 2016
P. Sbraccia et al. (eds.), *Clinical Management of Overweight and Obesity:
Recommendations of the Italian Society of Obesity (SIO)*,
DOI 10.1007/978-3-319-24532-4_11

progressively from 95.5 cm to 98.5 in all age groups [3]. On the other hand, in Europe, between 12.8 and 20.2 % of the men and between 12.3 and 25.6 % of the women older than 50 years are obese [4].

In Italy, considering a recent ISTAT report, a higher prevalence of overweight (46.4 %) and obesity (15.8 %) has been described in the group of individuals with age ranging from 65 to 74 years. [5]. Moreover, 30 % of the old subjects admitted to a nursing home were obese, and 30 % of them presented a body mass index (BMI) higher that 35 kg/m² [6]. Considering the progressive aging of population, it had been estimated an increase in the number of obese older adults up to 20.9 million in the USA and 32 million in the EU [7].

11.2   Clinical Evaluation of the Obese Older Subject

Obesity is a disease characterized by an excessive amount of adiposity associated with elevated health risk. Current guidelines suggest to use *BMI* as an index of adiposity and recommend the same cut-off values of BMI in the elderly as in younger adults [8]. However, BMI should be interpreted with caution in older ages, as BMI is a composite index of total body weight accounting for height, and aging may modify both the numerator (weight) and the denominator (height) of this index. Because of spinal deformity with thinning of the intervertebral discs as well as loss of vertebral body height due to osteoporosis, height may decline with age from 3 up to 5 cm. As a consequence, age-dependent height decline may itself induce a false BMI increase of 1.5 Kg/m² in men and 2.5 Kg/m² in women across aging despite minimal changes in body weight [9]. Further, body weight in old people reflects a higher amount of total fat because of the simultaneous progressive age-dependent loss of lean body mass (the so-called *sarcopenia*; see below). As a consequence, body fat percentage increases with age at every BMI, so that it is possible to hypothesize that the BMI thresholds used to categorize weight categories should be different in older than in younger ages.

Waist circumference has been proposed as a surrogate of adiposity and fat distribution in adults. The advantage of waist circumference over BMI is that it is relatively simple, useful for office assessment, independent of stature, and strongly related to both visceral and total fat. Measurement should be done at the level of the iliac crest by using a rigid tape with the patient standing and at the end of a normal expiration. Abdominal muscle tone decrease may determine underestimation of the amount of adiposity, or more realistically may determine some difficulty in the evaluation of waist circumference.

Waist circumferences cut-off points of 102 cm in men and 88 cm in women have been suggested for adults to indicate excess fatness. Using these cut-offs, a very large proportion of subjects aged 60 years and older have been judged to be affected by abdominal obesity, so that some researchers suggest that these cut-offs should be age specific [9].

11.3 Obesity and Mortality in the Elderly

The relationship between overweight and mortality in the elderly remains controversial. Andres et al. observed a *U-shaped* curve between BMI and mortality in old age, with age-related shift towards higher values of BMI associated with lower mortality [10]. A *J-shape* relation was actually observed in other studies. The possible explanation of these discrepancies might be found in the several confounding variables that should be taken into consideration when examining the association between obesity and mortality in the elderly. For example, there are variations across studies in the outcomes considered (total or specific mortality), in the confounders accounted for in the analysis (smoking, concurrent illnesses, weight changes), and in the length of the study follow-up [9]. In summary, since confounding effects accumulate over lifetime, it is difficult to accurately measure and account for all these factors. Also, since obesity acts on cardiovascular mortality in part through high blood pressure, dyslipidemia, or diabetes, aggressive treatment of these consequences of obesity may minimize the relationship between obesity and mortality in the elderly.

All together, the abovementioned confounding variables may be at least partially responsible for the *Obesity Paradox*, a term coined by Gruberg et al., who observed that patients with overweight or obesity had significantly lower in-hospital mortality and one year mortality than normal weight after percutaneous coronary intervention [11].

11.4 Clinical Consequences of Obesity in the Elderly

Obesity exacerbates the age-related *decline in physical function*. In cross sectional analyses, high values of BMI (>30 kg/m^2) in subjects aged 60 years or older have been shown to be related to functional impairment as measured by self-reported functional limitations in mobility, even considering different tests, such as time-up and go, stair climbing, and walking ability. Self-reported functional capacity, particularly mobility, is markedly diminished in overweight and obese compared to lean elderly adults [12]. Moreover, obesity has been shown to be a significant predictor of worsening in activity of daily living (ADL) in the elderly. Consecutively, older persons who are obese have also a greater rate of nursing home admissions than those who are not obese.

Obesity is also associated with fat deposition inside muscles, a known factor affecting muscle mass quality; this ectopic fat deposition has been shown to be an independent predictor of mobility limitation even after adjustment for demographic, lifestyle, and health factors. Finally, there is evidence that weight gain from adult to old ages is associated with impaired physical function and ADL disability in elderly subjects.

The *metabolic syndrome* (MetS) is more common in older than in younger subjects; its prevalence in the USA increases with aging, raising from about 4 % at the age of 20 years to almost 50 % at the age of 60 years. Similarly, in Italy 31.5 % of men and 59.8 % of women are affected by MetS.

Each cluster of MetS has been shown to be related to BMI and, in particular, body fat distribution also in the elderly [13]. Data from the Honolulu Heart Program suggest that obesity and high blood pressure continue to be highly correlated even in old age and that it may be possible to modify rates of hypertension by preventing weight gain. In both young and old adults, dyslipidemia, in terms of low HDL cholesterol and high serum triacylgerol levels, is associated with abdominal obesity. BMI and, in particular, indices of abdominal fat are related with greater risk of glucose metabolism disorders (both impaired fasting glucose and type 2 diabetes mellitus—DM) even in the elderly. A meta-analysis of 18 prospective studies, including subjects aged 18–80 years, showed that the relative risk of DM was 7.19 for obese persons and 2.99 for overweight subjects compared to those with normal weight. Interestingly, beside fat mass and visceral fat increase, even a reduction in peripheral fat, as evaluated by hip circumference decline, has been shown to be a predictor of diabetes in older ages. Not surprisingly the duration of obesity has a key role in the development of DM and has been shown to be a strong predictor of DM independently of current BMI.

Additionally, obesity is considered one of the most important risk factors for *osteoarthritis* (OA), especially for knee osteoarthritis. Prevalence of osteoarthritis increases in older ages in both sexes, together with the age-related increase in body weight [14]. A recent meta-analysis showed that being obese increases the risk of knee OA of 2.66 in the elderly. Obesity has been shown to be related also to psoriatic arthritis and increased risk of gout.

Age-related body composition changes are also related to the increase of *respiratory problems* in the elderly. Obese older men are particularly predisposed to develop shortness of breath and obstructive sleep apnea syndrome (OSAS). BMI is twice as strong as gender and fourfold stronger than age in predicting OSAS. Moreover, in a 30-year follow-up study age, baseline waist circumference as well as waist changes were the most powerful predictors of OSAS in old obese and normal weight men [7].

Urinary incontinence is more common in obese than in normal weight old subjects. This is particularly true for women in whom all types of incontinence (urge, stressor, or mixed) have been shown to increase linearly with BMI.

Being obese in older age increases the risk of breast *cancer,* as shown by a study including 300,000 women in which postmenopausal women with a BMI higher than 30 kg/m^2 showed an excess risk of 31 % of breast cancer than women with normal weight. Higher incidence of other cancers, such as pancreatic, uterine, cervical, colon, prostate, and gallbladder has been shown in older obese subjects.

A *U-shaped* association between BMI in midlife and *dementia* has been widely shown, with underweight and obesity as main risk factors for dementia. Association between increased BMI in midlife and neuronal and/or myelin abnormalities primarily in the frontal lobe as assessed by computed tomography has been reported.

In the elderly, a greater amount of adiposity often co-occurs with a decreased amount of muscle mass, a phenomenon called *sarcopenic obesity* (SO). Definition of SO should combine those of sarcopenia and obesity [15]. Sarcopenic obesity was defined by concurrence of sarcopenia (appendicular skeletal muscle mass divided by height squared less than two standard deviations below the sex-specific reference value for a young, healthy population) and high amount of fat mass (percentage of body fat greater than 27 % in men and 38 % in women or high values of BMI). Alternative definitions have been proposed later, some using cross tabulation of the highest quintiles of fat and lowest of fat-free mass, other using muscle strength instead of muscle mass. By using the abovementioned definitions, SO prevalence ranges between 4 and 22 % in men and women. Interestingly, irrespective of the definition used, SO prevalence increases with each decade of age. Actually, the criteria for the definition of SO are still not well standardized and raise some concerns, mainly because muscle quality, fat distribution indices, and evaluation of ectopic fat deposition are not taken into account in this definition. Some evidence indicates that when obesity and sarcopenia coexist in the elderly, they may act synergistically on the risk of developing multiple health adverse outcomes.

Despite the limitation due to the lack of a standardized definition, cross sectional and prospective studies support that SO subjects have higher risk of functional limitation, disability, frailty, poorer quality of life, longer hospitalization, and higher mortality compared with those with obesity or sarcopenia alone. In studies combining fat mass, as index of obesity, and strength, as index of sarcopenia, the association with physical function impairment is even stronger.

Thus, identification of old subjects with SO seems to be important in order to identify a group of subjects with a particular high risk of morbidity and mortality, which should be considered for treatment.

11.5 Treatment of Obesity in the Elderly

Numerous studies demonstrated that weight loss interventions even in people aged over 60 years lead to positive effects, such as significant improvements in glucose tolerance, reduced incidence of diabetes, reduced cardiovascular risk, improved functional and respiratory capacity, improvement of quality of life [7].

Nevertheless, as weight loss in old subjects may also induce some negative consequences, dieting and weight loss in elderly subjects should be engaged with particular attention to their effects on body composition. For example, lean body mass decrease ranges from 15 % of total body weight during a mild energy restriction to 50–70 % during semi-starvation [16] in adults, and these changes may determine the worsening of sarcopenia, with development of SO in elderly subjects [17]. For these reasons, strategies for management of obesity in the elderly should account for a multidisciplinary team, consisting of physicians, dieticians, therapists and exercise trainers, psychologists, caregivers.

Foremost, the *energy deficit* should be more moderate than in adults, up to 500 kcal under the daily energy expenditure, in order to reduce as much as possible the decline in lean mass.

A reasonable weight loss goal could be fixed at 5–8 % of the initial weight. Evidence shows that a moderate weight loss (nearly 5 %) in elderly women leads to a significant improvement in insulin resistance, fat distribution, muscle lipid infiltration and function, with a small decrease in appendicular lean tissue [18].

Additionally, the *protein intake* recommended in the elderly dieting should be 1.2 g/kg of ideal weight, adequately distributed over the meals, in order to counteract the possible blunted anabolic response in the elderly. Moreover, supplementation of essential amino acids, in particular leucine (6–8 g/day), has been proposed in order to increase protein anabolism and to decrease protein breakdown [7]. Optimal intake of specific micronutrients such as vitamin D, calcium, vitamins B6 and B12 should be achieved through adequate supplementation.

Adding *physical exercise* to the diet is mandatory in elderly subjects, as well as in adults. The combined effect of diet and exercise has been demonstrated to improve pain and functional status in people aged >60 years with radiographic evidence of osteoarthritis and self-reported physical disability [19]. The combined intervention (diet plus exercise) in a group of 107 obese frail elderly subjects followed for one year during a caloric restriction (500–750 kcal deficit) resulted more effective than the alone treatment diet or exercise in reducing the state of frailty, through achieving improvement in physical performance, functional status, and aerobic endurance capacity [17]. Moreover, a recent systematic review further confirmed that the association of diet and exercise resulted in a minor decrease of lean body mass compared to diet alone. Some debate still persists about the type of physical exercise to recommend during weight loss. Current data suggest that progressive resistance training, which stimulates protein synthesis and leads to muscle hypertrophy with increased muscle mass and muscle strength, combined with endurance training, which increases aerobic capacity, could be the optimal strategy to achieve metabolic improvements and to reduce functional limitations in the elderly [7]. Anyway, peculiarities of older ages should be considered when setting up physical activity programs.

Moreover, changing the lifestyle in older people, with modifications of the diet and with the attempt to counteract sedentary habits, is difficult because of the burden of disease; the frequent presence of isolation and loneliness, or institutionalization; the presence of sensory dysfunctions (impaired vision and hearing); and the frequent limited financial resources. For this purpose, behavioral therapy, including self-monitoring, social support, physical activity being a social activity as a group, relapse prevention, could be recommended even in older people.

Pharmacological Treatment The majority of the studies on pharmacological treatment of obesity does not consider older ages. A two-year randomized study conducted in the primary care setting on adults aged >65 years demonstrated that orlistat was as effective in older as in younger adults [7]. Orlistat is a lipase inhibitor that blocks the digestion and absorption of up to one third of the ingested fat, with an energy deficit of approximately 300 kcal/day. Main side effects of orlistat, such as flatulence, fecal incontinence, oily spotting, urge, steatorrhea, and abdominal cramps, occurring especially if high fat meals are consumed, should be carefully controlled during treatment. While liquid stools may counteract the typical constipation of the elders, this could represent a disabling problem particularly for those elders that have impaired sphincter function. Moreover, the absorption of fat soluble vitamins (A, D, E, K) may be reduced by orlistat, even though rarely below the limits of deficiency. Absorption of drugs could be also impaired if taken near the ingestion of orlistat, a problem that could be particularly frequent and dangerous in older ages, frequently characterized by polipharmacotherapy.

Anyway, it has been demonstrated that in elderly obese patients, orlistat, in combination with hypocaloric diet, produces more weight loss than diet alone, with no significant increase in adverse effects [20].

Bariatric Surgery (BS) Obesity management remains an important challenge in severely obese patients at any age. Bariatric surgery has been well established to be both safe and effective, although it remains a demanding procedure and applicable to a limited number of patients, especially they showed for the elderly. In a study conducted on 1339 elderly patients who underwent BS they showed, more comorbidity; longer lengths of stay; more postoperative pulmonary, hemorrhagic, and wound complications; and higher in-hospital mortality rates were observed in the older subjects [21]. Bariatric surgery is certainly not without potential morbidity and mortality, especially in the elderly, but in appropriately selected obese subjects could be lifesaving, although an increase in the number of bariatric procedures performed in the elderly, reaching 10 % of all bariatric operations performed at academic centers, has been observed. Moreover, it seems that the in-hospital mortality in BS in the elderly has improved so much that it is now even better than that of younger adults [22]. Although older adults seem to experience less weight loss, it seems that the surgical intervention could have potential benefits for these patients, as it has been observed a significant improvement in hypertension, diabetes, and, to a lesser extent, dyslipidemia in older patients undergoing BS; however, no data are available regarding the inflammatory profile of these patients [23]. All these observations concern short-term result of BS, so that long-term trials are needed to better evaluate the benefit of BS in aged obese patients.

References

1. Flegal KM, Carroll MD, Kit BK et al (2012) Prevalence of obesity and trends in the distribution of body mass index among US adults, 1999–2010. JAMA 307(5):491–497
2. Li F, Fisher KJ, Harmer P (2005) Prevalence of overweight and obesity in older U.S. adults: estimates from the 2003 Behavioral Risk Factor Surveillance System survey. J Am Geriatr Soc 53(4):737–739
3. Ford ES, Maynard LM, Li C (2014) Trends in mean waist circumference and abdominal obesity among US adults, 1999–2012. JAMA 312(11):1151–1153
4. Andreyeva T, Michaud PC, van Soest A (2007) Obesity and health in Europeans aged 50 years and older. Public Health 121(7):497–509
5. Micciolo R, Di Francesco V, Fantin F et al (2010) Prevalence of overweight and obesity in Italy (2001–2008): is there a rising obesity epidemic? Ann Epidemiol 20:258–264
6. Lapane KL, Resnik L (2005) Obesity in nursing homes: an escalating problem. J Am Geriatr Soc 53:1386–1391

7. Mathus-Vliegen EM, Obesity Management Task Force of the European Association for the Study of Obesity (2012) Prevalence, pathophysiology, health consequences and treatment options of obesity in the elderly: a guideline. Obes Facts 5(3):460–483
8. WHO (1997) Preventing and managing the global epidemic of obesity: report of the world health organization consultation of obesity. WHO, Geneva
9. Zamboni M, Mazzali G, Zoico E et al (2005) Health consequences of obesity in the elderly: a review of four unresolved questions. Int J Obes (Lond) 29:1011–1029
10. Andres R, Elahi D, Tobin JD et al (1985) Impact of age on weight goals. Ann Intern Med 103:1030–1033
11. Gruberg L, Weissman NJ, Waksman R et al (2002) The impact of obesity on the short-term and long-term outcomes after percutaneous coronary intervention: the obesityparadox? J Am Coll Cardiol 39:578–584
12. Vincent HK, Vincent KR, Lamb KM (2010) Obesity and mobility disability in the older adult. Obes Rev 11:568–579
13. Han TS, Tajar A, Lean ME (2011) Obesity and weight management in the elderly. Br Med Bull 97:169–196
14. Villareal DT, Apovian CM, Kushner RF et al (2005) Obesity in older adults: technical review and position statement of the American Society for Nutrition and NAASO, The Obesity Society. Am J Clin Nutr 82:923–934
15. Zamboni M, Mazzali G, Fantin F et al (2008) Sarcopenic obesity: a new category of obesity in the elderly. Nutr Metab Cardiovasc Dis 18:388–395
16. Ballor DL, Katch VL, Becque MD et al (1988) Resistance weight training during caloric restriction enhances lean body weight maintenance. Am J Clin Nutr 47(1):19–25
17. Villareal DT, Chode S, Parimi N et al (2011) Weight loss, exercise, or both and physical function in obese older adults. N Engl J Med 364(13):1218–1229
18. Mazzali G, Di Francesco V, Zoico E et al (2006) Interrelations between fat distribution, muscle lipid content, adipocytokines, and insulin resistance: effect of moderate weight loss in older women. Am J Clin Nutr 84:1193–1199
19. Messier SP, Loeser RF, Mitchell MN et al (2000) Exercise and weight loss in obese older adults with knee osteoarthritis: a preliminary study. J Am Geriatr Soc 48(9):1062–1072
20. Mathys M (2005) Pharmacologic agents for the treatment of obesity. Clin Geriatr Med 21(4):735–746
21. Varela JE, Wilson SE, Nguyen NT (2006) Outcomes of bariatric surgery in the elderly. Am Surg 72(10):865–869
22. Gebhart A, Young MT, Nguyen NT (2014) Bariatric surgery in the elderly: 2009–2013. Surg Obes Relat Dis 11(2):393–398
23. Caceres BA, Moskowitz D, O'Connell T (2015) A review of the safety and efficacy of bariatric surgery in adults over the age of 60 (2002–2013). J Am Assoc Nurse Pract 27(7):403–410

Multidimensional Assessment of Adult Obese Patient Care and Levels of Care

12

Barbara Cresci, Mario Maggi, and Paolo Sbraccia

12.1 Multidimensional Assessment

Obesity is a complex disease that requires a complex approach, multi- and interdisciplinary, and possibly always tailored to the needs of each patient. According to the phenotyping of the patient, a possible pathway should be selected, involving first of all the primary care services. The next level of intervention will feature specialized outpatient clinics, including different professional figures (i.e., a multidisciplinary team possibly consisting of internist/endocrinologist, nutritionist/dietitian, psychiatrist/psychologist, physiotherapist/graduate in physical education). These professionals could be supported, where necessary, by other specialists for specific comorbidities. A "team building" action is therefore necessary to make possible a good coordination of the work. The intervention provided by the specialist could finally be realized, depending on the clinical functional and psychological-psychiatric patient conditions, as semi-residential or residential, in specialized structures (acute care or rehabilitation). In some cases, as indicated in the specific chapter, bariatric surgery could be suggested, again as part of a process of global and lasting patient care.

B. Cresci (✉)
Section of Diabetology, Careggi University Hospital, Florence, Italy
e-mail: b.cresci@dfc.unifi.it

M. Maggi
Department of Experimental and Clinical Biomedical Sciences,
Andrology and Sexual Medicine Unit, University of Florence, Florence, Italy
e-mail: m.maggi@dfc.unifi.it

P. Sbraccia
Department of Systems Medicine, Medical School, University of Rome "Tor Vergata",
Rome, Italy

Internal Medicine Unit and Obesity Center, University Hospital Policlinico Tor Vergata,
Rome, Italy
e-mail: sbraccia@med.uniroma2.it

© Springer International Publishing Switzerland 2016
P. Sbraccia et al. (eds.), *Clinical Management of Overweight and Obesity:
Recommendations of the Italian Society of Obesity (SIO)*,
DOI 10.1007/978-3-319-24532-4_12

12.2   Levels of Care

12.2.1 Programs Provided Directly by Primary Care Services (General Practitioners—GPs, Pediatricians, Outpatient Nutritional Prevention)

The primary care services, and in particular the GPs, are tasked to screen the patients; to identify predisposing factors; to monitor and evaluate their evolution; to evaluate the general clinical, functional, and psychological conditions; to assess motivation to change; to implement corrective lifestyle measures; to use drug therapy to treat possible complications; to address patients, where necessary, to specialized structures where the patients could have access to multidisciplinary integrated care. The role of primary care remains fundamental in defining with the patient an appropriate totally shared and rational therapeutic strategy.

The Cochrane Collaboration evaluated [1] the effectiveness of educational interventions at GP level, concluding that recommendations cannot yet be drawn up concerning their effectiveness and the best way to implement them but signaling a likely more effective intervention if a team nutritionist/doctor/nurse is available in supporting GPs. More recently [2], the US Preventive Services Task Force has confirmed, based on the evidence of the literature, the importance of interventions aimed at weight loss provided in primary care; it particularly emphasizes the efficacy and safety of behavioral treatments for weight loss in the maintenance phase.

The most important problem for the GP could be to find enough time to spend with these patients, within a complex system of care that must take into account all kinds of diseases, including emergencies.

12.2.1.1   Proposal for the Intervention of GPs with Obese Patients: Clinical Diagnosis

		Timing
Anthropometric parameters	Height	Baseline
	Weight	Baseline, monthly during the therapeutic process, then in half-year maintenance phase
	BMI calculation	
	Waist circumference	
Clinical history	History of the weight	Baseline with periodic check
	Nutritional history (including alcohol)	
	Smoking habits	
	Exercise habits/level of physical activity	
	Medications	

		Timing
Evaluation of comorbidities	Heart rate	Baseline with periodic check
	Fasting glucose (OGTT if necessary)	
	Lipid profile (total cholesterol, HDL, LDL, triglycerides)	
	Total testosterone (males)[a]	
	Symptoms suggestive of cardiorespiratory complications (dyspnea, angina, obstructive sleep apnea syndrome)	
	Bone/joint diseases and disabilities	
	Symptoms suggestive of an eating disorder	
Psychological status	Level of anxiety and depression	Baseline with eventual periodic check
	Quality of life	
	Motivation to change	

[a]The relation between obesity and hypogonadism is well known and widely supported by clinical studies performed in the general population. In particular, the European Male Ageing Study, a multicenter clinical trial involving more than 4000 subjects over 40 years of age from eight different countries, has demonstrated that testosterone levels decrease with age, but obesity is able to anticipate the age-related reduction in testosterone levels of about 15 years.

The GPs could possibly find it difficult, in some situations, to devote so much time to the care of these patients. In this case, they will have to study possible alternative strategies (for instance, within consortia of GPs), before sending the patient to a second level structure.

12.2.1.2 Proposal for the Intervention of GPs with Obese Patients: Management, Therapeutic Intervention, and Monitoring

Intervention	See before for timing
Lifestyle counseling	
*Nutritional education	
*Correction of inactivity	
Eventual pharmacotherapy	

Once rated the excess weight, quantified the risk and the presence of associated diseases and psychological status, the primary care services will:

1. Work on motivation where there is no willingness to enter a treatment
2. Propose a therapeutic intervention characterized by:
   - * Information for a correct lifestyle (generic or, where possible, custom tailored) (see specific Chaps. 2 and 3)
   - Prescription of drugs to treat associated diseases
   - Periodic check of results and adherence to therapy

3. Work together with specialized second level structures:
    *   When the degree of obesity is severe (BMI $\geq$ 35)
    *   In presence of important comorbidities (BMI $\geq$ 30 with comorbidities and/or disability)
    *   In presence of an eating disorder (BED) or suspicion of concomitant psychiatric illness

    Anyway, even if the primary care services should send the patient to a specialist, it would be appropriate/recommended that the GPs could collaborate with the specialists in long-term monitoring, whatever the patient characteristics is, interacting in particular when the degree of obesity is higher and the framework of associated diseases are more severe [3].

    As part of the monitoring, the contribution of primary care services/GPs includes:
    *   Evaluation of the anthropometric variables (weight, BMI, waist circumference)
    *   Assessment of vital signs (PA, FC)
    *   Evaluation of associated diseases
    *   Pharmacovigilance (also in case of pharmacotherapy firstly prescribed by a specialist)

    As part of the monitoring, these situations should suggest sending the patient to the specialist:
    *   Poor adherence to therapy
    *   Important side effects of treatment
    *   Clinical worsening of associated diseases

12.2.1.3 Treatment of Obesity at the Primary Care Service Level: How Long

Baseline BMI levels	Weight reduction goal
25–29.9 kg/m^2	5–10 % in 6 months
30–34.9 kg/m^2	5–15 % in 6–12 months
35–39.9 kg/m^2	15–>20 % in 12 months
	In patients with a history of frequent treatment failures and/or with a very low level of motivation, a therapy focused on weight maintenance should be the treatment to be proposed while waiting to be able to start weight loss therapy.

12.2.2 Programs Supplied in Specialist Outpatient Settings

In the development of a clinical care management team for patients suffering from obesity, it would be desirable to develop networks including the presence of both primary care services and specialist facilities. The latter, structured in outpatient settings, should possibly have interdisciplinary teams consisting of physicians with expertise and experience in the evaluation and treatment of eating disorders and obesity (internist, psychologist/psychiatrist, bariatric and plastic/reconstructive surgeon, dietitian, physiotherapist, graduate in physical education where possible). Although effective integration of skills within the team could be desirable, if this is not possible, in some cases, these skills could be found in other external structures. Nevertheless, it is necessary that these skills should concern the treatment and management of obese patients.

Therapeutic education must be the guide throughout the course of treatment, and all the professionals should be involved, within their peculiar competences, in the treatment planning (see Chap. 4).

The possibility to set up groups of education for patients requiring the intervention of different professional roles, or in order to support patients, may be taken into account. Even the European Guidelines provide "an evidence-based approach, but at the same time allowing flexibility to the clinician in those areas where at the moment evidence is not available."

Time/patient: at least 60 min for the first visit and 20–30 min for the controls of each professional

12.2.2.1 Proposal of Activities for Specialist Outpatients: Clinical Diagnosis

1. Physical examination, with particular attention to:
   - Weight
   - Height
   - BMI
   - Waist circumference
   - Blood pressure
   - Heart rate
   - Examination targeted to the complications of obesity known or suspected
2. Accurate History:
   - Family history: excess weight, metabolic disorders, and cardiovascular
   - Weight history: age of onset of obesity and weight history
   - Pharmacological and dieting history: anorectic/antiobesity drugs, other drugs, types of diet followed in the past
   - Nutritional history: eating habits and frequency of meals
   - Evaluation of previous or current medical history suggestive of secondary causes of excess weight (e.g., genetic, drugs, endocrine disorders)
   - Evaluation of other possible determinants of obesity (e.g., psychosocial factors, chronic stress, smoking cessation)
   - Current and previous physical activity
   - Evaluation of eventual present or past diseases, commonly associated with excess weight
   - Smoking habits
   - Alcohol consumption

- Snoring at night
- Daytime hypersomnia
- Evaluation of osteoarticular and motor function
3. Blood chemistry with particular attention to:
   - Fasting blood glucose, HbA1c
   - Lipid profile (total cholesterol, HDL, LDL, triglycerides)
   - Uricemia
   - Liver enzymes
   - TSH
   - Total testosterone (males) (any other endocrinological investigation only in case of clinical suspicion)
4. Evaluation of body composition
   - Bioimpedance (recommended technique)
   - (DEXA) (although it is the gold standard, it is not recommended in clinical practice and it has to be reserved for clinical trials)
   - Indirect calorimetry (where available)
5. Evaluation of the psychological state
   - Attitude of the patient relative to his weight (to assess how the patient lives his physical appearance; investigate if he feels significantly limited in his social life, work, and sex to avoid situations that he would live with discomfort because of its weight)
   - Expectations towards weight loss and motivation to change
   - Evaluation of the possible presence of an eating disorder
   - Evaluation of the possible presence of depression and other mental disorders, including clinically significant pathological addictions

	Frequency/timing	Notes
Clinical examination	Every control visit (physician, dietitian, or nurse)	Weight (BMI), waist circumference
Blood chemistry	If needed (medical decision)	
Body composition	Every control visit	Physician or dietitian
Comorbidities	Every control visit (physician)	
Evaluation of the psychological/psychiatric state	Baseline (+ in case of significant change in weight)	General and specific psychopathology (eating disorders, body image, quality of life)

12.2.2.2 Proposal for the Specialist Intervention in Obese Outpatients: Management, Therapeutic Intervention, and Monitoring

Obesity treatment for specialist outpatients must include:

- Therapeutic education (see specific chapter) – the real needs of patients should be recognized, and on that basis we will attempt to correct the misconceptions on nutrition and physical activity, to improve not only the knowledge but also the skills, to train self-management, physical activity, control of simple clinical parameters (blood glucose, blood pressure), moments of stress, and anxiety by encouraging compliance with therapy.

- Nutrition for the purposes of caloric restriction (see specific chapter), on the basis of estimated energy expenditure also based on physical activity (assessed with BIA results) – prior to prescription (energy input, micro- and macronutrients) and in agreement with the patient, the dietitian will develop the dietary pattern that, according to the rules of a healthy diet, will have to meet the needs and desires of the patient as much as possible.

- Reduction of physical inactivity (see specific chapter) – after medical evaluation (physiatrist, cardiologist, pulmonologist), the patient will start a program of physical reconditioning and/or rehabilitation (motor, cardiac, or respiratory), which will then be managed by the physiotherapist and/or graduate in physical education according to the patient's needs. Depending on the ability of the patient, directions on how to start (or increase) the motor activity will be given. The program will be as personalized as possible on the basis of the possibilities and the clinical conditions of the patient, suggesting a gradual increase of the intensity/frequency of the exercise. At each visit, patient adherence to the program must be checked.

- Any drug treatment for obesity and/or drugs for eventual complications

- Possible management of psychiatric comorbidity (see specific chapter)

Since obesity is a chronic disease, it is necessary to have a proper follow-up (to minimize the risk of drop-out and loss of compliance of the patient) and a continuous supervision is needed to prevent the recovery of weight, to monitor the risk of disease and treat comorbidities. Because the follow-up could be considered appropriate, a certain frequency of checks, during the phase of weight loss, of one visit per month, and during the maintenance phase, of one visit every three–four months, should be provided. The frequency of checks will be adjusted if necessary based on the presence and severity of comorbid conditions.

Intervention	Who	Frequency	How
Therapeutic Education	All operators i.e. Psychologist/ Psychiatrist + physician, dietitian, physiotherapist and/or graduate in physical education	Weekly	Individually Group (max 10 patients)
Nutritional intervention	Prescribed by the physician and elaborated by the dietitian	Reevaluation every control visit	Pounded diet plan, diet therapy based on portioning, suggestions on food style modification (eventually food diary)

Intervention	Who	Frequency	How
More active lifestyle	Experts (graduate in physical education, physiatrist)	Baseline + verify any change at every control visit	Give information on how to start (or increase) physical activity Exclude the presence of absolute contraindications together with the physician Personalize the exercises based on the possibilities and clinical condition of the patient, suggesting a gradual increase of the intensity/frequency of the exercise. Evaluate at every control visit patient adherence to the program
Drug prescription and pharmacovigilance	Physician		
DCA and/or psychiatric comorbidities management	Psychologist and/or Psychiatrist	Medical decision, based on the needs of the individual patient	Face-to-face or group intervention based on the needs of the individual patient

12.2.2.3 Specialist Intervention in Obese Outpatients: How Long

Regarding weight reduction, the same criteria identified for interventions delivered at a local GP could be applied.

BMI levels	Weight reduction Italian GL	Weight reduction European GL
30–34.9 kg/m^2	5–10 % in 12 months	5–15 % weight loss in 6 months or prevention of weight regain
35–39.9 kg/m^2	5–10 % in 12 months	Consider also higher rates of weight loss (>20 %)
40 kg/m^2 or more	10–15 % in 12 months	

The criteria for long-term success [4] are represented by:

- Maintenance of weight loss
- Prevention and treatment of comorbidities

As mentioned above, 12 months of follow-up represent the minimum period to assess the long-term effectiveness of a program for weight loss. However, where possible an evaluation at longer times would be indicated to evaluate the best strategies for prevention in patients who tend to relapse afterwards.

Higher levels of treatment in poor responders	After a maximum follow-up of 12 months, in case of absent or not sufficient results in the treatment of obesity and its complications and in case of BMI $\geq$ 35 kg/m^2 (in presence of comorbidities) or BMI $\geq$ 40 kg/m^2 (in presence of significative quality of life reduction), consider the possibility to send the patient to higher levels of treatment: Intensive interdisciplinary rehabilitation in Day Hospital Intensive interdisciplinary rehabilitation for inpatient Bariatric surgery, according to the criteria and the appropriate indications defined by the current Guidelines (see specific chapter) considering the degree of self-efficacy of the patient, the level of motivation, and the risk–benefit ratio.

12.2.3 Programs Provided by Inpatient Specialists

BMI $\geq$ 45 kg/m^2 even without known comorbidities
BMI $\geq$ 35 kg/m^2 in presence of comorbidities
BMI $\geq$ 40 kg/m^2 already treated as outpatients without significant results

12.2.3.1 Acute Care

The hospital stay in acute care regimen for patients suffering from obesity, especially high-grade obesity, in places suitably fitted in terms of adequate instruments, structures, organizations and equipped with the appropriate expertise and technical assistance (see relative chapters of this Document), is one of the cornerstones of the clinical management of the obese patient. Admission to acute care regimen can be considered appropriate:

(a) Regardless of the obesity level, in presence of medical conditions that put the patient at risk of life in the short term
(b) In cases of intermediate and high-grade obesity given the presence of comorbid conditions in clinical imbalance and requiring an intensive care which is not feasible in the outpatient setting or at least not feasible with times and effectiveness required
(c) In cases of high-degree obesity with suspected or proven comorbidity or significant disability requiring for its diagnosis and for the definition of the appropriate therapeutic-rehabilitative intervention investigations not possible in outpatient settings or complex multidisciplinary evaluations

Regarding case (a), it is appropriate that the patient with high-grade obesity should be addressed, possibly during the process of triage exerted by the operators of emergency-urgency territorial services, to highly specialized hospitals within the region or at least that the patient could be transferred there, once his clinical conditions have been stabilized. As for cases (b) and (c), hospitalization generally occurs in an Internal Medicine ward. The assessment involves process indicators, appropriateness indicators, and outcome indicators.

A week-long hospitalization can also precede the rehabilitation program as a result of an acute event or planned on the basis of the comorbidity and clinical risk level (SSA-RMNP-O $\geq$ 30) [5]. This hospitalization has the purpose to make the clinical condition more stable and to perform a multidimensional interdisciplinary assessment which may allow a more effective rehabilitation.

12.2.3.2 Metabolic-Nutritional-Psychological Rehabilitation in a Semi-Residential or Residential Setting

In recent years, it has become more evident the relationship, independently of the presence of chronic pathologies, between BMI and various degrees of disability. According to the World Health Organization, obesity is the sixth leading cause of disability worldwide. The Consensus SISDCA SIO-2009 has also proposed an instrument for evaluating the appropriateness of the access to metabolic-nutritional rehabilitation: the SIO form on Appropriateness of Metabolic Nutritional Psychological Rehabilitation of the obese patient (SSA•RMNP•O) (6; www.SIO-obesita.org).

In particular, in the SISDCA SIO-2009 Consensus (24) we can read: "The intensive rehabilitation is a crucial node in the service network when:

1. The level of severity and/or medical and/or psychiatric comorbidity is high.
2. The impact on disability and quality of life of the patient is important.
3. Interventions to be implemented become numerous, and it is appropriate—for clinical and economic reasons—to concentrate them quickly in a coordinated project.
4. Previous programs with lower intensity have not yielded the desired results, and the risk for the patient's health tends to increase".

The program of Metabolic-Nutritional-Psychological Rehabilitation of obese patients (see specific chapter) integrates, in an interdisciplinary approach, a nutritional intervention, a motor/functional rehabilitation program, a therapeutic education and focused short psychotherapeutic interventions, a nursing rehabilitation.

Flow chart

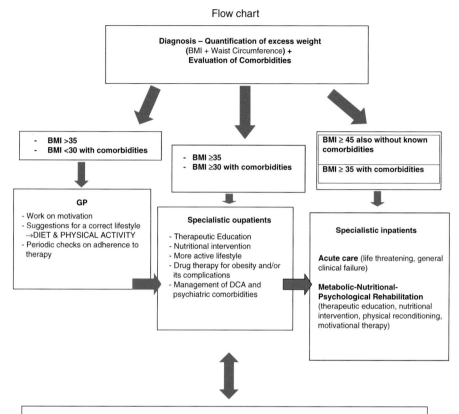

References

1. The Counterweight Project Team (2008) Influence of body mass index on prescribing costs and potential cost savings of a weight management programme in primary care. J Health Serv Res Policy 13(3):158–66
2. Erin S, LeBlanc ES, O'Connor E, Whitlock EP, Patnode CD, Kapka T (2011) Effectiveness of Primary Care–Relevant Treatments for Obesity in Adults: A Systematic Evidence Review for the U.S. Preventive Services Task Force. Ann Intern Med 155:434–44
3. Centro Studio e Ricerca sull'obesità (2003) Università degli Studi di Milano. Obesità, Sindrome Plurimetabolica e Rischio Cardiovascolare. Rischio cardiovascolare. Consensus sull'inquadramento diagnostico-terapeutico
4. Centre for public health excellence at NICE (UK); National collaborating centre for primary care (UK). Obesity: The prevention, identification, assessment and management of overweight and obesity in adults and children [Internet]. London: National institute for health and clinical excellence (UK); 2006 Dec. (NICE Clinical guidelines, No. 43.) Available from: http://www.ncbi.blm.nih.qov/books/NBK63696/
5. Donini LM et al (2010) Consensus. Obesity and eating disorders. Indications for the different levels of care. An Italian Expert Consensus Document. Eat Weight Disord 15:1–31

Treatment Algorithm of Patients with Overweight and Obesity: SIO (Italian Society of Obesity) Treatment Algorithm (SITA)

13

Ferruccio Santini, Luca Busetto, Barbara Cresci, and Paolo Sbraccia

In approaching the treatment of obesity, three major caveats, specific of this complex disease, need to be taken into consideration in order to avoid hyper simplification.

First, obesity definition is based on an index, body mass index (BMI), that has two major limitations: it is not a measure of fat mass, and it does not include measures of regional fat depots. These limitations are well acquainted by the scientific community that is struggling to find out ways to overtake BMI.

Second, the development of comorbidities, or complications as we prefer to define them, present in the vast majority of obese patients is not always linearly correlated, for the reasons specified above, with BMI. Many variables contribute to their manifestation beyond the degree of obesity: duration of disease, age, sex, fat distribution, genetic background, the degree of mechanical disability, etc.

SIO (Italian Society of Obesity) Treatment Algorithm COnsensus Panel (SITA-COP): Paolo Sbraccia, Luca Busetto, Barbara Cresci, Fabrizio Muratori, Enzo Nisoli, Ferruccio Santini, Roberto Vettor.

For the SIO (Italian Society of Obesity) Treatment Algorithm COnsensus Panel (SITA-COP)

F. Santini
Obesity Center, Endocrinology Unit, University of Pisa, Pisa, Italy

L. Busetto
Department of Medicine, University of Padua, Padua, Italy

B. Cresci
Section of Diabetology, Careggi University Hospital, Florence, Italy

P. Sbraccia (✉)
Department of Systems Medicine, Medical School, University of Rome "Tor Vergata", Rome, Italy

Internal Medicine Unit and Obesity Center, University Hospital Policlinico Tor Vergata, Rome, Italy
e-mail: sbraccia@med.uniroma2.it

© Springer International Publishing Switzerland 2016
P. Sbraccia et al. (eds.), *Clinical Management of Overweight and Obesity: Recommendations of the Italian Society of Obesity (SIO)*,
DOI 10.1007/978-3-319-24532-4_13

Third, treatment options are now quite few. Their indications should take into account the severity of obesity together with the presence and severity of complications and age, in order to grade interventions from therapeutic lifestyle changes to bariatric surgery.

In order to provide a staging system able to help clinicians in phenotyping obese patients, beyond BMI, Sharma and Kushner [1] developed the so-called EOSS (Edmonton Obesity Staging System) composed of the following five stages:

0. No apparent obesity-related risk factors (e.g., blood pressure, serum lipids, fasting glucose, etc., within normal range), no physical symptoms, no psychopathology, no functional limitations and/or impairment of well-being
1. Presence of obesity-related subclinical risk factors (e.g., borderline hypertension, impaired fasting glucose, elevated liver enzymes, etc.), mild physical symptoms (e.g., dyspnea on moderate exertion, occasional aches and pains, fatigue, etc.), mild psychopathology, mild functional limitations, and/or mild impairment of well-being.
2. Presence of established obesity-related chronic disease (e.g., hypertension, type 2 diabetes, sleep apnea, osteoarthritis, reflux disease, polycystic ovary syndrome, anxiety disorder, etc.), moderate limitations in activities of daily living and/or well-being.
3. Established end-organ damage such as myocardial infarction, heart failure, diabetic complications, incapacitating osteoarthritis, significant psychopathology, significant functional limitations, and/or impairment of well-being.
4. Severe (potentially end-stage) disabilities from obesity-related chronic diseases, severe disabling psychopathology, severe functional limitations, and/or severe impairment of well-being.

The EOSS was then validated as a system able to identify patients at increased mortality risk who therefore deserve more clinical and therapeutic attention [2].

We took advantage of this now well-established staging system to develop a therapeutic algorithmic chart (Fig. 13.1) that includes BMI, age, and EOSS stages. At each intersection, a color code identifies the proposed preferred treatment option. Obviously, treatment options are not mutually exclusive but have to be intended as additive (e.g., a patient eligible for bariatric surgery should continue to follow therapeutic lifestyle changes and, if needed, pharmacotherapy).

We certainly believe that chronic diseases such as obesity have to be faced with flexibility and understanding; any treatment option should be thoroughly explained to patients while sharing with them our analysis of the rationale and cost–benefit ratio behind any proposed treatment, treatment that ultimately has to be tailored to the single patient. However, any algorithm that may help clinicians in their delicate choices is always welcome. We deeply hope this would be the case for our chart.

In this chapter, we will not indicate any level of evidence or strength of recommendation since this is based on an expert opinion ground and evidence is at the moment insufficient.

Treatment Algorithm of Patients with Overweight and Obesity

EOSS	BMI < 30	BMI 30-35	BMI 35-40	BMI >40	Age (years)
STAGE 0					> 60
					< 60
STAGE 1				S	> 60
					< 60
STAGE 2				S	> 60
					< 60
STAGE 3			S	S	> 60
					< 60
STAGE 4					> 60
					< 60

lifestyle intervention

pharmacological therapy
(In patients with T2DM, is indicated the use of antidiabetic medications that have additional actions to promote weight loss, such as GLP-1 analogs).

bariatric surgery

rehabilitation (physical, neurological, cardiopulmonary, psychiatric)

S   surgery to be considered in selected cases with favorable risk/benefit profile

Fig. 13.1 Treatment algorithm chart that take advantage of the EOSS (Edmonton Obesity Staging System, see text and Ref. [1]). At each intersection a color code identify the proposed preferred treatment option. Obviously, treatment options are not mutually exclusive but have to be intended as additive

References

1. Sharma AM, Kushner RF (2009) A proposed clinical staging system for obesity. Int J Obes (Lond) 33(3):289–295
2. Kuk JL, Ardern CI, Church TS, Sharma AM, Padwal R, Sui X, Blair SN (2011) Edmonton Obesity Staging System: association with weight history and mortality risk. Appl Physiol Nutr Metab 36(4):570–576

Index

A
Abdominal obesity
  dyslipidemia, 148
  MetS, 147–148
  sarcopenic obesity, 148
  waist circumferences, 146
Abdominal ultrasound, 62–63
Activities of daily life/instrumental
    activities of daily life
    (ADL/IADL), 87
Activity of daily living (ADL), 147
Adherence therapeutic, 38–39
Adiposity
  early rebound, 136
  obese older subject, 146
Adjustable gastric banding
  single bariatric procedure, 75
  surgical techniques, 64
Adolescent obesity
  diet therapy, 16
  health gain, 138
  overweight/obesity, 139
  therapeutic programs, 138, 139
Adult obese patient
  care, levels of
    inpatient specialists, 161–163
    primary care services, 154–156
    specialist outpatient settings, 156–161
  multidimensional assessment, 153
Aerobic exercise
  definition, 26
  physical activity, 135
  vigorous-intensity, 26
Alcohol
  naltrexone, 50
  weight-maintenance, 15
α-melanocyte-stimulating hormone
    (α-MSH), 50
Amino acids, 49, 150

Anorexia nervosa (AN)
  grazing, 103
  weight suppression, 101
Antibiotic prophylaxis, 64, 124
Anti-obesity
  drug treatment, 46
  orlistat, 47
Attention-deficit/hyperactivity disorder
    (ADHD), 108

B
Bariatric/plastic-reconstructive surgery
  outcomes improvement, 84
  rehabilitative pathway, 90
Bariatric surgery (BS)
  adolescents, 58–59
  adults
    BMI, 57, 58
    contraindications, 58
    guidelines, 56
  choice of bariatric operation,
    criteria, 72
  drug treatments, 73
  DSM-5 criteria vs. DSM-IV
    provisional criteria, 103
  elderly obesity, 151
  follow-up, 73–74
  grazing, 103
  intragastric balloon, 72–73
  metabolic-nutritional-psychological
    rehabilitation, 163
  multidimensional assessment, 153
  NES, 104
  nutritional prescriptions, 73
  patients aged over 60 years, 60
  patients with BMI 30–35 kg/m^2,
    60–61
  preoperatory evaluation, 62–63

© Springer International Publishing Switzerland 2016
P. Sbraccia et al. (eds.), *Clinical Management of Overweight and Obesity:
Recommendations of the Italian Society of Obesity (SIO),*
DOI 10.1007/978-3-319-24532-4